SECOND EDITION

POCKET NOTES ON neonatology

SECOND EDITION

Editor

Dr Mark W Davies, MB, BS, FRACP, DCH
Senior Staff Specialist in Neonatology, Grantley Stable Neonatal Unit, Royal Brisbane and Women's Hospital, Brisbane, Queensland
Associate Professor of Neonatology, Department of Paediatrics and Child Health, The University of Queensland, Brisbane, Queensland

Co-editors

Dr David W Cartwright, MB, BS, FRACP, BSc
Director of Neonatology, Grantley Stable Neonatal Unit, Royal Brisbane and Women's Hospital, Brisbane, Queensland

Dr Garry DT Inglis, MB, BS, FRACP
Staff Specialist in Neonatology, Grantley Stable Neonatal Unit, Royal Brisbane and Women's Hospital, Brisbane, Queensland

CHURCHILL LIVINGSTONE
ELSEVIER

Sydney Edinburgh London New York Philadelphia St Louis Toronto

ELSEVIER

Churchill Livingstone
is an imprint of Elsevier

Elsevier Australia
(a division of Reed International Books Australia Pty Ltd)
Tower 1, 475 Victoria Ave, Chatswood, NSW 2067
ACN 001 002 357

National Library of Australia Cataloguing-in-Publication Data

---

Davies, Mark W.
Pocket notes on neonatology.

Includes index.
ISBN 978 0 7295 3832 9 (pbk.).

1. Neonatology - Handbooks, manuals, etc. I. Cartwright, David W. II. Inglis, Garry. III. Title.

618.9201

Publishing Editor: Sophie Kaliniecki
Developmental Editor: Sunalie Silva
Publishing Services Manager: Helena Klijn
Editorial Coordinator: Lauren Allsop
Edited by Teresa McIntyre
Proofread by Andy Whyte Media Services
Index by Max McMaster
Cover, internal design and typesetting by Toni Darben
Printed by 1010 Printing International Ltd.

Preface

This second edition of *Pocket Notes on Neonatology* has been substantially updated with a large amount of revised and new material. However, it still remains the only genuinely pocket-sized book of its kind.

The information contained in this book was originally designed to guide junior medical officers and nursing staff who care for infants admitted to the intensive and special care nurseries at the Royal Brisbane and Women's Hospital (RBWH). This second edition has been revised with a far wider readership in mind, with many sections now more general. Despite that, however, many of the ways of doing things described in this book may differ from those used elsewhere, and the reader is encouraged to always check how things are done in their nursery and not to rely only on the information in this book.

In publishing this book we aim to facilitate the care of the newborn infant. However, this information alone is not sufficient to guide health professionals making decisions about care of the newborn infant. That requires careful evaluation of a number of different factors, including information and judgment about needs, resources, values, the applicability of and quality of evidence, and an understanding of the nature and basis of disease and its treatment.

Mark W Davies
David W Cartwright
Garry DT Inglis

Acknowledgments

We would like to acknowledge and thank the following for their help with preparing this book:
Kirsteen Mackay
Donna Bostock
Steve Withers
Jeremy Robertson
Luke Jardine.

Contents

Abbreviations

BE	base excess
BP	blood pressure
BSL	blood sugar level
BW	birth weight
$[Ca^{2+}]$	calcium ion concentration
$[Cl^{-}]$	chloride ion concentration
CI	confidence interval
CMV	conventional mechanical ventilation
CNS	central nervous system
CP	cerebral palsy
CPAP	continuous positive airway pressure
Cu	copper
CVL	central venous line
CXR	chest X-ray
DAT	direct antibody test
EBM	expressed breast milk
ELBW	extremely low birth weight
EOGBSD	early onset GBS disease
ETT	endotracheal tube
FBC	full blood count
FiO_2	fraction of inspired oxygen
GA	gestational age
GBS	group B *Streptococcus*
[Hb]	haemoglobin concentration
HbF	fetal haemoglobin
HFV	high-frequency ventilation
HIE	hypoxic-ischaemic encephalopathy
HMD	hyaline membrane disease
HR	heart rate

IA	intra-arterial(ly), intra-arterial line
ICC	intercostal catheter
IM	intramuscular(ly)
IPPV	intermittent positive-pressure ventilation
IV	intravenous(ly), intravenous line
IVH	intraventricular haemorrhage
$[K^+]$	potassium ion concentration
Mg	magnesium
$[Na^+]$	sodium ion concentration
NG	nasogastric
Nsaline	Normal saline (0.9%)
P	phosphorus
$PaCO_2$	partial pressure of carbon dioxide in arterial blood
PaO_2	partial pressure of oxygen in arterial blood
PCR	polymerase chain reaction (test)
PEEP	positive end expiratory pressure
PIP	peak inspiratory pressure
PN	parenteral nutrition
$[PO_4^{3-}]$	phosphate ion concentration
PVE	periventricular echogenicity
PVL	periventricular leucomalacia
RBC	red blood cell
SBR	serum bilirubin level
SpO_2	oxygen saturation
STAT	immediately
UAC	umbilical arterial catheter
UVC	umbilical venous catheter
V/Q	ventilation–perfusion
VLBW	very low birth weight
Zn	zinc

CHAPTER 1

Infection control — hand hygiene

David Cartwright and Mark Davies

Hand washing

Hand washing remains the most effective method of preventing the spread of organisms from ourselves to babies, and hence between babies. Such organisms usually transfer from a baby to adult hands to another baby, and probably via nursery equipment.

- If you have any infected areas around your nails or fingers, you should not work with patients until they have cleared.
- Do not wear watches or jewelled rings while caring for babies. Plain rings only are acceptable. Jewelled rings have many crevices which cannot be cleaned effectively, and often have sharp edges which can scratch.
- Always wash hands and forearms (up to the elbows) before touching any patient for any reason. Wet hands and forearms first, then apply the antibacterial solution — this minimises skin reactions, and aids adequate spread and anti-bacterial activity.

  We recommend the antibacterial solution Microshield T (containing triclosan); see note below. Chlorhexidine-based hand washes are also common.
- Antiseptic alcohol-based hand rub may be available for use at the bedside on occasion, for rapid entry only. It should **not** be used if you have just come from outside the nursery, nor if your hands have been soiled by any previous handling. If used, hands and forearms must be

well covered, and it must then be allowed to dry before entering the cot.

Examples include Hexol with chlorhexidine and ethanol, or Microshield hand gel with ethanol and moisturisers.

Note: The introduction in 1991 of Microshield T (containing triclosan) for hand washing in the intensive care (ICN) and special care nurseries (SCN) at the Royal Brisbane and Women's Hospital was responsible for the virtual disappearance of MRSA (methicillin-resistant *Staphylococcus aureus*) colonisation — instead of being endemic, it is now very rare and sporadic. Babies are also washed in Microshield T in the ICN.

Maintaining hand hygiene

After washing, the hands should not touch **anything** else before handling the baby. Charts, paperwork, monitors, ventilators, the outsides of incubators, etc are all regarded as 'dirty' — not to be touched after hand washing before touching a baby.

- Be particularly careful not to touch your face, hair, etc; nor the patient's chart, observation sheets or cot surrounds.
- Go directly from the sink to the baby.
- Open incubator doors with the backs of your hands.
- On ward rounds, do not lean on cots or equipment.
- Picking up the patient's observation records one after another on a ward round is a good way to transfer germs rapidly around the nursery. Can you do a ward round without picking up every baby's observation sheets?
- Avoid touching monitors or ventilators and going back into a baby's incubator. If it is really essential to cancel a monitor alarm, do it with the back of a knuckle, which is then unlikely to touch a baby before the hands are washed again.
- If called to the telephone or elsewhere, always wash again before resuming caring for a baby. Telephones are great places for transmitting germs from one adult to

another — mouth to mouthpiece to hands, handset to hands, and so on.

Hygiene guidelines — equipment and procedures

- Wash your stethoscope between babies. A simple good habit is to rub the tubing and bell of your stethoscope while hand washing, when you have handwashing solution on your hands, then wipe the stethoscope with the paper towel used to dry your hands. Alternatively, wipe your stethoscope over with an alcohol wipe (isopropyl alcohol). Remember these precautions are even more important, although more difficult, in busy and crowded times.
- Clean all other items that move from cot to cot, e.g. ultrasound probes should be wiped with an alcohol wipe between patient uses.
- Remember that any time we break skin integrity, there is a risk of making a colonising organism into an infecting organism. Be very careful that:
  - all procedures involving making a hole in the skin are necessary
  - all skin preparation is carefully done
  - time is given for skin preparation solutions to dry before inserting a needle. If using iodine, wait two minutes. If using alcoholic chlorhexidine, wait for natural drying.
- If you are having difficulty with a procedure with multiple attempts, get someone else to do it — we all have bad days.
- Be very sparing of requests for capillary gases — the glass capillary tube is not sterile. Why make a hole in the skin and then rub a non-sterile glass rod in it?

CHAPTER 2

Resuscitation

David Cartwright, Garry Inglis and Mark Davies

Assessment

Many physiological changes occur when a fetus becomes hypoxic and/or ischaemic in utero.

After delivery, varying degrees of cardiorespiratory depression may be observed. An attempt to quantify this, made by Dr Virginia Apgar, is now called the **Apgar score** — a score of 0 to 2 is assigned to each of 5 variables. This score in itself does not help you in making resuscitation

Sign \ Score	0	1	2
Heart rate	absent	<100	>100
Respiratory effort	absent	poor or irregular	good regular breaths or lusty cry
Reflex irritability (with nasal or pharyngeal suction)	no response	grimace	cough or sneeze
Muscle tone	flaccid	poor tone with some flexion of arms or legs	good tone with spontaneously flexed arms and legs which resist extension
Colour	blue all over	pink with blue extremities	pink all over

decisions, nor does it predict outcome with any degree of accuracy, but the components of it are useful in your assessment of the baby.

Heart rate (HR)

Heart rate is helpful in three situations:

1. Is it present in the totally apnoeic atonic baby? Persisting apnoea and hypotonia despite adequate HR may be due to brain injury, a congenital neuromuscular disorder, or sedation secondary to maternal medication.
2. Is it persistently low in the pink and vigorous baby? Whilst persistent bradycardia is almost always indicative of continuing hypoxia — check that you are delivering oxygen effectively, that your endotracheal tube (ETT) is correctly positioned, and that the chest is moving adequately — very uncommonly it is due to heart block.
3. As a useful guide to successful resuscitation — it rises rapidly.

Other considerations

- Special consideration in resuscitation must be given to babies born through meconium-stained liquor (page 10), diaphragmatic hernia, upper airway obstruction and pulmonary hypoplasia.
- Remember that an unexpected need for resuscitation (the unexpectedly 'flat' baby) can be a sign of infection. This is often overlooked in assessing a baby's infection risk (see page 107).
- Hypo- or hyperthermia is common following resuscitation. Both are potentially harmful and should be avoided.
- In a prolonged resuscitation it is usually desirable to obtain vascular access. The simplest and fastest way to achieve this is to insert a catheter into the umbilical vein (UV) — see page 19 for description. This can then be used for administration of drugs (including fluids), and for obtaining blood samples.

Drugs

Drugs used in neonatal resuscitation are few:

- **Oxygen** — given via mask or ETT.
  Whether air, 100% oxygen or some lower concentration of oxygen is used at the start of resuscitation is controversial — the policy will differ from unit to unit. Regardless, adequate inflation of the lungs is the most essential aim of resuscitation.
- **Adrenaline** — via UV (can also be given via IV/ETT).
- **Fluid for volume expansion** — via IV/UV (see note below).
- **Sodium bicarbonate** — via IV/UV (see note below).
- **Naloxone** — via IV/UV/IM (see note below).

Note: Evidence for the roles of fluid for volume expansion, bicarbonate and naloxone in resuscitation is weak. They should rarely be required.

Basic equipment

The following is a basic list of equipment that should be available for neonatal resuscitations:

- A firm surface
- Overhead radiant warmer
- Warm towels
- Suction equipment
- Oxygen supply
- Resuscitation bag or T-piece device; masks; ETTs
- Laryngoscopes
- Meconium suction device
- Feeding/gastric tubes
- UV catheterisation kit
- Syringes and needles
- Saline, drugs.

Resuscitation flow diagram

See opposite. In general, this scheme is consistent with both the Neonatal Resuscitation Program run by the American

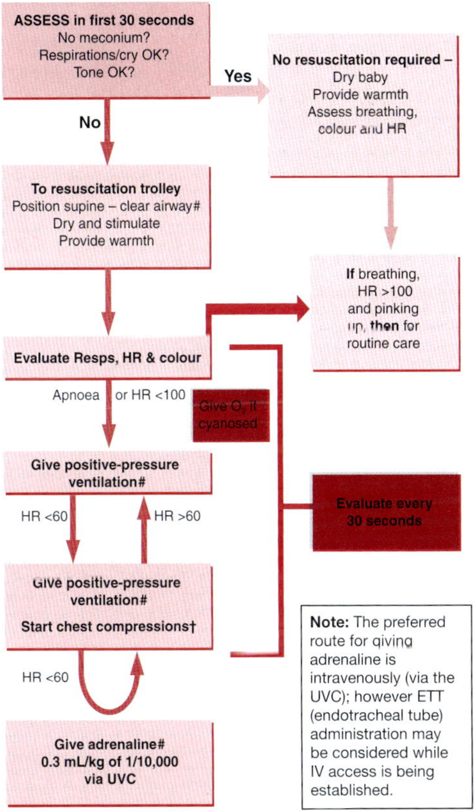

Figure 2.1 Resuscitation flow diagram

HR = heart rate; Resps = respirations; UVC = umbilical venous catheter.

Endotracheal intubation needs to be considered here.

† Give 3 chest compressions and 1 breath every 2 seconds
1, 2, 3, breath..1, 2, 3, breath…
(i.e. 90 compressions and 30 breaths per minute).

Heart Association and the American Academy of Pediatrics [Kattwinkel J, ed. Textbook of neonatal resuscitation. 5th edn. Chicago: American Academy of Pediatrics and American Heart Association; 2006]; and the Australian Resuscitation Council Neonatal Guidelines revised February 2006 [available at www.resus.org.au/].

When to stop unsuccessful resuscitation

Resuscitation should stop when a baby has been asystolic for 10 minutes despite adequate resuscitation (especially adequate lung expansion).

Resuscitation equipment

T-piece resuscitation device (e.g. Neopuff)

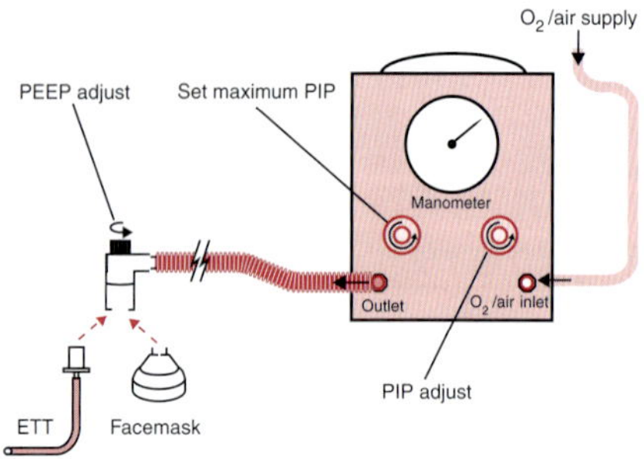

Figure 2.2 T-piece resuscitation device
ETT = endotracheal tube

Flow-inflating bag

(aka CPAP bag, anaesthetic bag)
Dependent on a flow of gas into the bag.

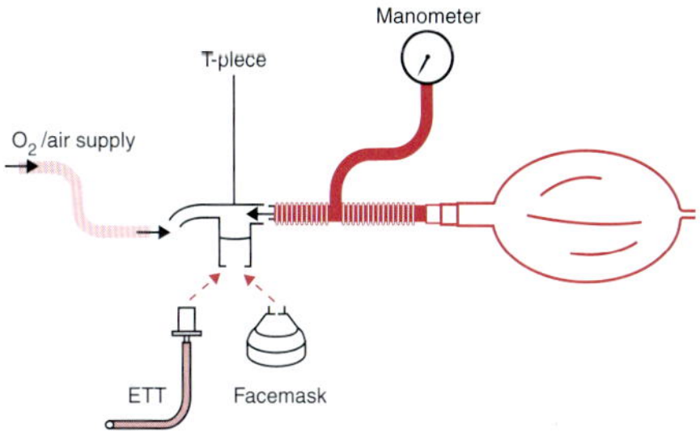

Figure 2.3 Flow-inflating bag
ETT = endotracheal tube

Self-inflating bag

Reinflates automatically after squeezing for each breath. Can be used without a flow of gas into it.

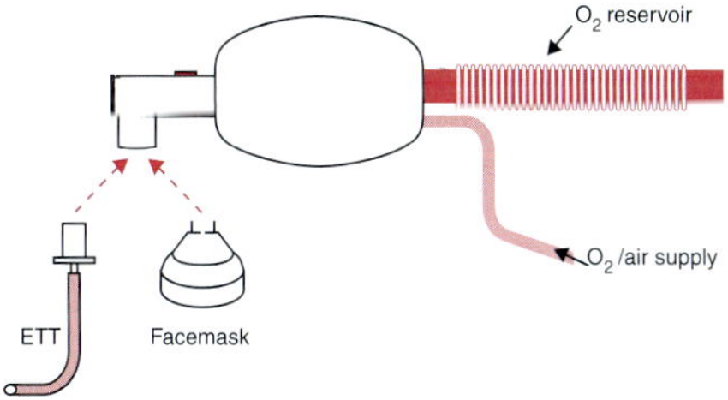

Figure 2.4 Self-inflating bag
ETT = endotracheal tube

Meconium-stained liquor

Meconium staining of the liquor is reported to occur in approximately 12% of labours. In only a small proportion of these, the fetus or a newborn infant may aspirate some meconium into his/her lungs, causing subsequent respiratory distress. Mostly when aspiration occurs, it is because of accompanying asphyxia, reaching the stage of gasping respirations prior to delivery. Aspiration of meconium does not occur with normal fetal breathing movements. Therefore when there is no asphyxia, the fetus is extraordinarily unlikely to ever aspirate meconium.

The **management** of the fetus and baby revolves around two principles:

- The prevention of aspiration of meconium from the pharynx after delivery.
- The removal of already aspirated material from the airway.

This management is effected by the following steps:

1 Member of the paediatric medical staff (e.g. registrar, house officer, resident) to be present in labour ward/birth suite.

2 After delivery, if the baby is active and vigorous and establishes its own respirations, it should be allowed to do so, as attempted clearance of meconium in such a baby has been shown to make no difference to the outcome.
Vigorous = strong respiratory efforts, good muscle tone and HR >100 bpm.

3 If there is any respiratory depression, the baby should be taken immediately, without stimulation, to the resuscitation trolley for assessment and management by paediatric staff.

4 Paediatric staff look at the pharynx and suction any meconium.

5 If continued respiratory depression is present, the baby should be intubated. For a term baby, a size 3.5 ETT should be used. The trachea is then suctioned by sucking directly on the ETT. This is achieved using a metal

T-piece (which is normally used to deliver oxygen) or a meconium aspirator (Fig 2.5).

— Attach the sucker to the usual oxygen delivery connection of the metal T-piece, or to the narrow end of the meconium aspirator, and place a finger/thumb over the open end of the connector.

— Suck on the ETT with low suction for a few seconds and then continue sucking while the ETT is removed.

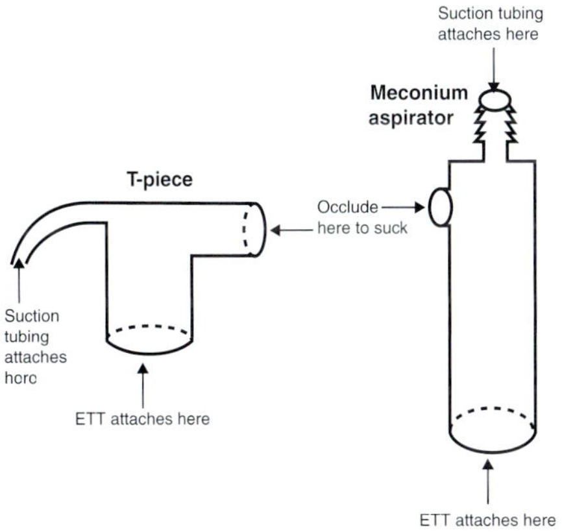

Figure 2.5 Equipment for sucking on ETTs
ETT = endotracheal tube

> **!** Suctioning of the trachea should not be performed using a sucker passed down through the ETT. Direct suctioning of the trachea using a sucker without an ETT is not advised. Saline lavage is also not advised.

6 Repeat suction as in step 5 until meconium is no longer recovered from the trachea, or until the baby's condition dictates that resuscitation should now proceed in the usual way. It is unusual to need to repeat this suction more than twice.

7 Babies who then develop any respiratory distress or have abnormal chest sounds should be observed in the Special Care or Intensive Care Nursery. Babies with meconium aspiration are at high risk of pulmonary hypertension (see page 60).

Based on recent evidence from randomised controlled trials, the major resuscitation councils around the world no longer recommend routine suctioning of the baby's nose and mouth prior to delivery of the shoulders.

CHAPTER 3

Procedures

David Cartwright and Mark Davies

Skin disinfection — general principles

Whenever we break the skin integrity of a baby, we run the risk of making a skin-colonising organism into an infecting organism. Risks are minimised:

1. by limiting the number of times skin integrity is breached
2. by ensuring adequate skin preparation whenever it is necessary to breach skin integrity.

Skin preparation solutions

- Alcoholic chlorhexidine may be used routinely as a skin preparation solution for procedures. Aqueous chlorhexidine is recommended for extremely low birth weight (ELBW) infants in the first few days of life.
  Alcohol wipes (isopropyl alcohol) may be used for heel-prick blood tests, arterial 'stabs' and intramuscular/ subcutaneous injections. In addition, use iodine for central venous line insertions before the alcoholic chlorhexidine.
- Skin disinfecting solutions take time to work.
  Iodine and chlorhexidine need about 2–3 minutes skin contact time for optimal disinfection; alcohol about 30–60 seconds, or until the alcohol evaporates.
- **Never** allow too much alcoholic chlorhexidine to sit on a baby's skin, especially that of ELBW infants.
- Skin preparation solutions should always be allowed to dry of their own accord. They should never be 'wiped

off'. A minute or two of waiting may save a week or two of antibiotics! — a good trade-off.

Pain relief

The options for analgesia during procedures are:

- none
- swaddling
- cuddling and facilitated tucking
- breast feeding
- skin-to-skin contact
- non-nutritive sucking
- oral sucrose
- IV narcotics.

Vascular access

Peripheral intravenous (IV) cannula

- A 24G cannula is adequate for almost all neonatal applications.
- This is a two-person procedure.
- Use a sterile disposable dressing pack.

Technique

1. Wear sterile gloves.
2. Lay a sterile paper towel (or drape) under the limb.
3. Cleanse the insertion site thoroughly with a suitable skin preparation solution, allowing this to dry before inserting the cannula.
4. Try not to touch the insertion site at all.
5. Reapply skin preparation solution to the skin if multiple attempts at insertion are necessary.
6. Use a new cannula for each new attempt. The person inserting the IV should not open new cannulae themselves, nor get new ones out of a drawer.
7. If the task looks or becomes too difficult, get someone more experienced.

Remember, every new hole in the skin increases the infection risk and the pain for the baby.

Umbilical arterial catheter (UAC) insertion

> If in a Level 2 nursery **do not** put a UAC in an ELBW or critically ill baby without consulting your Level 3 regional centre, and **never** use the second umbilical artery once attempted cannulation of the first umbilical artery has been unsuccessful. Vascular access for these babies in the first week of life is critical.

General preparation

- Inserting a UAC is a two-person procedure — the assistant holds and monitors the baby during the procedure.
- Use a full sterile technique.
- We suggest direct consultant supervision for infants <28 weeks GA and <1000 g BW.

Most nurseries will have a pre-prepared catheter insertion tray set up. In addition you will need the following items, all sterile:

- a cord tie
- a 5 mL syringe
- heparinised Normal saline (Nsaline, 0.9%) (10 units/mL)
- catheter — use size 5FG catheter for babies ≥1500 g, 3.5FG for <1500 g
- scalpel blade
- 3-way tap
- suture.

Insert the 3-way tap into the catheter and fill with heparinised Nsaline.

> If inserting both an umbilical artery (UA) and an umbilical vein (UV) line, insert the UA line first, then the UV line. Tie in the UV line first, then the UA line. (See page 21.)

Technique for UAC insertion

1 If working in an incubator, 'line' the insides of the entry doors first with a sterile dressing towel each to minimise the risk of unsterilising your hands on entry to the cot.

2 Cleanse abdomen, cord and cord clamp: use alcoholic chlorhexidine unless baby is <1000 g BW; if so use aqueous chlorhexidine. Then place a cord tie around the base of the cord to prevent ooze from the umbilical vein. The top of the cord tie should be level with the skin line (Fig 3.1).

3 Be careful not to let any skin preparation solution (especially alcoholic chlorhexidine) spill down the sides of the abdomen — a small infant lying in this for even a short time may receive 2nd or 3rd degree burns over the flanks and buttocks.

> **!** **Never** use so much alcoholic chlorhexidine that it sits for prolonged periods of time in contact with the baby's skin, and **never** let it dribble down the sides of the baby so that the baby is lying in contact with alcohol-soaked drapes, nappies or bedding.

4 Cut cord cleanly (with a single slicing motion) about 1 cm above the skin line. Discard cord clamp and forceps used to hold clamp.

5 Use fine-toothed forceps to hold the stump near the vessel to be cannulated.
Some use artery forceps to do this, or place a suture through the upper part of the stump to hold it.

6 Identify the vessels (usually 2 arteries and 1 vein) — the arteries are smaller with thicker walls and sit proud of the cut surface; the vein is larger with a loose, thin wall.

7 Dilate the artery carefully with iris forceps.

8 Insert catheter to the correct distance:
— use the shoulder tip to umbilicus distance as a guide: measure from the tip of the left shoulder to the bottom of the umbilicus and put the catheter in this distance
— or use the 'ready reckoner' tables on pages 166–8.

9 Make sure you can aspirate blood back.

The number of different methods used to secure umbilical catheters is almost limitless. Best to learn what they do in your local intensive care nursery and do it. Our scheme is outlined below — it works well.

10 Place a purse-string suture around the stump (not the skin) and secure the catheter (Figs 3.1 and 3.2).
We use chromic-gut, as it grips the catheter well and if any is left behind after catheter removal it will dissolve away.

11 The first knot on the catheter should be 0.5 to 1 cm above the purse-string knot.

12 The knots on the catheter should be tight enough that the catheter cannot be pulled through the knots, but not so tight that they occlude the catheter lumen — check that you can still aspirate blood back.

13 Attach infusion line (with pressure transducer). An X-ray is required to check position.

14 An acceptable position for the tip is T6–T12. If it is lower than T12, pull back to L3–L4. Do not leave at L1–L2.

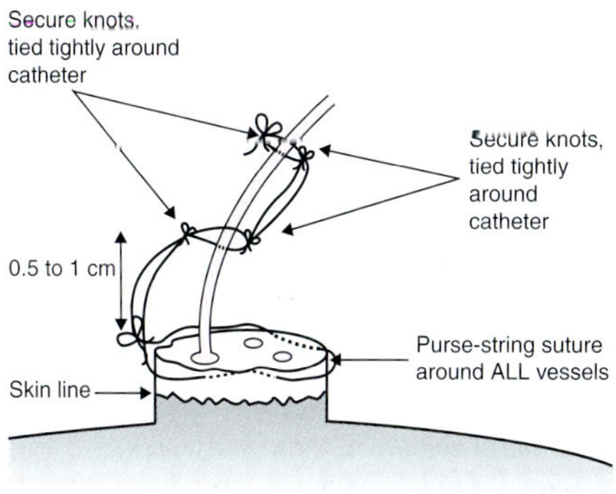

Figure 3.1 Suturing an umbilical catheter — side view

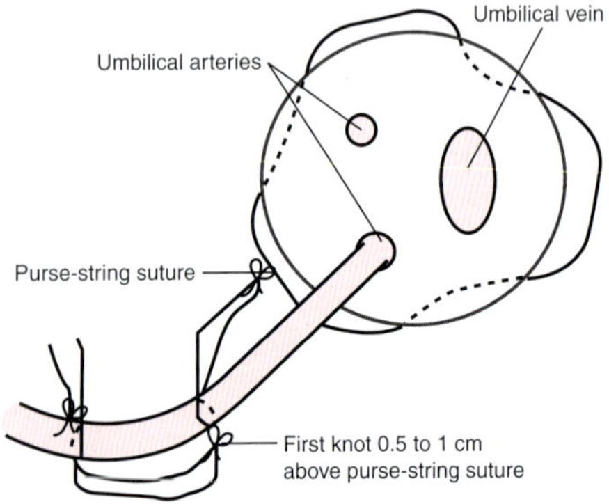

Figure 3.2 Suturing an umbilical catheter — top view

15 Now arrange more permanent strapping of the catheter. There are numerous ways of strapping the catheter and each neonatal unit will have their own method. We suggest sandwiching the catheters between two strips of tape along the abdominal wall and up the catheter. (This is similar to taping intercostal catheters — see Fig 4.8 on page 52.) Apply a transparent, bio-occlusive, polyurethane dressing (such as Bioclusive, Tegaderm, Opsite) to the abdominal skin so that the tape is stuck to this and not directly to the skin.

16 Make sure you have taken the cord tie off.

17 Check that lower limb perfusion is OK.

18 Usually UACs are left in situ for a maximum of 10 days.

Notes on UA infusions

- Standard UA infusion is Nsaline or 10% dextrose with 1 unit/mL of sodium heparin (NaHeparin).
- Parenteral fluids, including Na^+ and Ca^{2+}, can be administered through these lines, and antibiotics can also be given.

- Boluses of $NaHCO_3$ (sodium bicarbonate) may be given slowly (<1 mmol/min — total dose should not be given over less than 5 minutes).
- Boluses of Ca^{2+} should only be given with great care — you must take all responsibility for the potential complications.
- Vasodilating drugs such as tolazoline and prostaglandin may be given through UA lines. Vasoconstricting drugs such as dopamine should not, and neither should potentially particulate material such as blood or platelets (fresh frozen plasma/albumin are OK). Indomethacin is never given via an UA.

Umbilical venous catheter (UVC) insertion

Technique and equipment as for UAC insertion, page 15.

> **!** If inserting both an umbilical artery (UA) and an umbilical vein (UV) line, insert the UA line first, then the UV line. Tie in the UV line first, then the UA line. (See page 21.)

General preparation

- Prime the catheter with heparinised saline (10 units/mL).
- Use size 5FG catheter for babies ≥1500 g, 3.5FG for <1500 g. Use a dual lumen catheter if <1000 g or critically ill.

Technical points

1. The UV is usually readily identified and normally requires minimal or no dilatation. A blunt probe might help — point it towards the head as the course of the umbilical vein is directly cephalad from the umbilicus. The vein runs just beneath the skin immediately above the umbilicus, and the catheter or probe can often be felt there to confirm its position.
2. You can also use this course to your advantage if you need to stem haemorrhage, by placing your finger or a folded gauze square firmly above the umbilicus rather than directly pressing on the umbilicus, which will be end-on to the UV.

3 Insert catheter to correct depth:
   — 5–6 cm for babies <1000 g, 8–10 cm for large babies
   — some like to use the lower sternum to umbilicus distance as a guide: measure from the bottom of the sternum to the bottom of the umbilicus and put the catheter in this distance
   — or use the 'ready reckoner' tables on pages 166–8.
4 If you meet resistance before you have reached the desired distance, it is unlikely that you are through the ductus venosus into the inferior vena cava/right atrium (IVC/RA, Fig 3.3).
5 The catheter should only ever be left in a position where blood is easily drawn back into the catheter.
6 Place a purse-string suture around the stump (not the skin) and secure the catheter in similar fashion to that described for a UAC (page 17 and Figs 3.1 and 3.2). Attach infusion line. An X-ray is required to check position.
7 The best tip position is at the IVC/RA junction, which is around T8–T9, at the bottom of the heart at the level of the diaphragm.
   — If it is lower than T9, it is not usually through the ductus venosus. A catheter should not be left in this

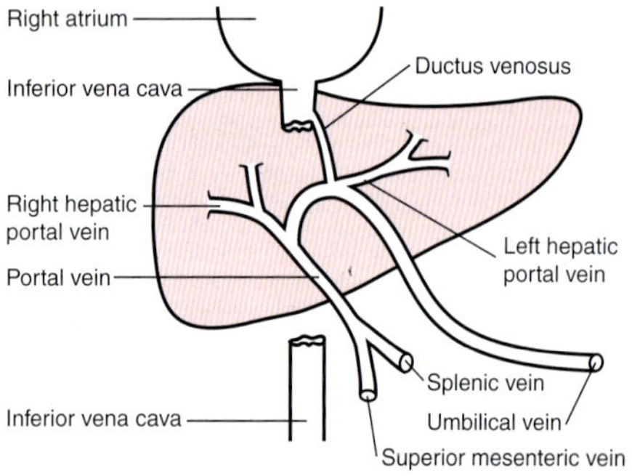

Figure 3.3 Schematic diagram of the umbilical vein anatomy

position for more than a few hours (unless vascular access is critical and problematic) and should only be used for saline or dextrose infusion and urgent antibiotics/blood products; using it for parenteral nutrition or inotropes should be avoided.

— If the catheter tip deviates over to the left or right within the liver shadow on X-ray, in one of the hepatic portal veins, it should be removed completely, or pulled back until the catheter sits vertically alongside the spine (umbilical vein) if considered critically needed.

8 Usually UVCs are left in situ for a maximum of 7 days.

Notes on UV catheters

- UV catheters tend to migrate inwards over the first day or two of life, and a repeat X-ray is wise to review the position. It is not uncommon to need to pull the catheter back 1 cm or so the day following insertion. Presumably the course of the vein straightens as the abdomen fills with gas.
- On the other hand, if the baby begins with marked abdominal distension which is relieved, the catheter tip may also migrate inwards.
- Perforation of the right atrial wall is a potentially fatal complication of UV catheters (and silastic percutaneous central lines).
  - If a baby with a UVC in place deteriorates rapidly and without immediate explanation, cardiac tamponade should be thought of and looked for — try aspirating the catheter, transillumination, CXR, cardiac echo.
  - If tamponade from a large pericardial effusion is strongly suspected or is diagnosed, aspirate it with an IV needle passed under the xiphisternum and directed postero-laterally to the left.

Securing both a UAC and a UVC

1 If both UA and UV catheters are inserted at the same time, insert the UA first, then the UV. Suture the UV first, then the UA.

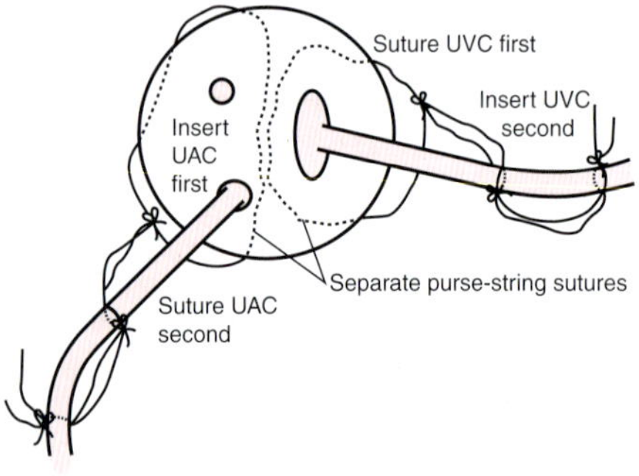

Figure 3.4 Suturing in two umbilical catheters — top view
UAC = umbilical arterial catheter; UVC = umbilical venous catheter

Reason: you often need to trim back the umbilical stump during insertion of a UA line, and this is difficult if a UV line is in place already. Also, the UV line will slip back very readily — take your eyes off it for a moment and it will be a few cm out from where you think you left it, so tie it first, and always recheck its position just before tightening the knot.

2. Tie the two catheters separately, as they are often removed or adjusted separately (Fig 3.4). Place two purse-string sutures in the stump around the vessels and catheters as shown in the diagram above.

Peripheral silastic central venous line (CVL) insertion

We recommend that this procedure is limited to consultant or 'attending' neonatologists and/or senior registrars or fellows.

Preparation

- Use a full sterile technique (sterile gown, gloves, mask).

- Cleanse the insertion site with iodine (left on the skin for at least 2 minutes) and then with alcoholic chlorhexidine (allowed to dry).
- Drape around the insertion site with a sterile window drape or four drapes arranged appropriately. The drapes should give you a large sterile surface to work from (i.e. next to the insertion site).
- The procedure is easier with the incubator side open, but this cannot be done if the cot temperature required is >35.5°C, as the baby will then become cool. If the cot side is open, be careful not to obstruct the warm airflow inside the cot.
- For minimal disturbance to the baby, observe these principles;
  - — Use one limb only for one attempted insertion.
  - — Limit yourself to 4 skin holes in that limb.
  - — If not in the vein within half an hour, stop and call on someone more experienced.

Technique

The procedure is simple: see vein; put needle in vein; thread catheter up needle.

1. Use medial arm veins by preference — if you use the cephalic vein you will often have difficulty getting the catheter past the shoulder region where the cephalic meets the axillary vein.
2. Insert the catheter the appropriate distance — a little too far is better than not far enough. Always ensure that you can freely and repeatedly withdraw blood into the catheter when it is in the position where you intend to leave it.
3. If there are no distance markers on the catheter you will need to measure (with a sterile tape measure) how much catheter remains outside the baby and subtract from 30 cm (for a 30 cm catheter). Then lay the tape measure over the presumed course of the vein this distance from the insertion site. Aim to have the catheter tip approximately 1–2 cm above the lower end of the sternum.

4 Cover the insertion site with a transparent, bio-occlusive, polyurethane dressing (such as Bioclusive, Tegaderm, Opsite). Do not coil any catheter under this dressing as this may lead to the catheter inadvertently advancing further into the vein.

5 The end of the catheter is then secured to an arm board.

6 After taping the catheter in, we always X-ray to confirm tip position with an injection of contrast (e.g. Isovue 300, 0.5 mL) — aim to be still slowly injecting while the X-ray is being taken. This allows identification of the tip of the CVL, as a blush of contrast will be seen as it leaves the tip; it will also show that infusate flows readily from the catheter tip. Aim to have the tip in the superior vena cava (SVC) or IVC, or where they enter

In a recent audit of our practice (2186 catheters) the following principles were identified as being important in the overall success of our use of percutaneous central venous lines [See: Cartwright DW. Central venous lines in neonates: a study of 2186 catheters. Arch Dis Child Fetal Neonatal Ed 2004;89:F504–F508.]

1 Inserted by experienced staff (e.g. consultant or senior registrar).
2 Aim to insert too far and pull back away from vessel walls.
3 Never leave a catheter where it does not easily and repeatedly withdraw blood during the insertion procedure.
4 ALWAYS inject with radio-opaque contrast for X-ray examination (if you don't inject it, you don't know where the tip is).
5 Be actively injecting during X-ray examination to see contrast coming from the end of the catheter.
6 Sterile technique for insertion, and for line changes (3 times/week).
7 No drug injections — catheter used for parenteral nutrition only.
8 Antifungal prophylaxis of oral and topical nystatin.
9 Cover insertion site with bio-occlusive dressing and leave undisturbed. No coils of catheter under dressing.

the RA. Any large vein will be OK. Some units will never leave a CVL tip in the heart.

Notes on CVLs

- Infants who have a CVL in situ should be commenced on oral and topical nystatin. [This policy was introduced at the Royal Brisbane and Women's Hospital in 1980 after a spate of systemic candidal infections in very low birth weight infants. From 1 January 1984 to 31 December 2001, 2044 CVLs were inserted, with septicaemia in 80 (2.4/1000 line-days). Only 4 cases of septicaemia were due to candida (0.2% of lines).]
- The parenteral nutrition solution and line should be changed three times per week (M,W,F) using a full sterile technique.

Peripheral intra-arterial (IA) line insertion

The technique is similar to that for IV cannula insertion.

- A 24G cannula is adequate for almost all neonatal applications.
- Wear sterile gloves.
- Assistant to hold limb while 'prepping' so that all of skin to be touched is disinfected.
- Make a sterile field using two sterile dressing towels.
- Reapply skin preparation solution for multiple attempts.
- The standard IA infusion is Nsaline or $^{1}/_{2}$NSaline with 2 units/mL of NaHeparin. Run at 0.5–2 mL/hr. **Never** give anything else via an IA line.

Specimen collection

Arterial blood gas 'stabs'

1. An alcohol wipe (isopropyl alcohol) is suitable skin preparation — allow the skin to dry.
2. Use a pre-heparinised syringe with a 25G needle.
3. Do all your feeling around to locate the artery before skin preparation, and try then to make the actual technique 'no touch' after wiping with the alcohol wipe.

4 Insert the needle, bevel upwards, into the artery and aspirate. If electrolytes are to be measured, aspirate slowly as haemolysis may occur during rapid withdrawal up a 25G needle, giving spuriously low [Na^+] and high [K^+].
5 Have pressure applied by someone else after sampling.

Sampling arterial catheters

1 Wash your hands. Hand preparation solutions alone are not adequate. Remember that this procedure, like breaching skin integrity, runs risk of taking colonising organisms and introducing them into the baby as infecting organisms.
2 Take a 2 mL syringe and a pre-heparinised 1 mL blood gas syringe. The 2 mL syringe should be inside its sterile wrapper so that its tip does not touch anything.
3 Hands should be washed again after syringe preparation, and before entering the cot. Wear gloves (they do not need to be sterile — they are to protect you from blood contamination, not to protect the baby from you).
4 Open incubator doors with the backs of your hands.
5 Wipe the 3-way tap clean with an alcohol wipe.
6 Ensure the tips of syringes do not come into contact with any surfaces during the procedure.
7 Remove and discard the 2 mL syringe that is already on the 3-way tap.
8 Use the new (clean and empty) 2 mL syringe to clear the line of at least 1.6 mL of fluid and blood. Turn the stop-cock to the 45° position — so all 3 'taps' are off. Replace this syringe into its original packet.
9 Change syringes and aspirate blood into the 1 mL blood gas syringe — 0.1 mL for an arterial blood gas (ABG). (0.6–0.8 mL for ABG plus electrolytes ± bilirubin if the sample is to be sent to the lab.) Remove bubbles.
10 Never reinject any blood from the blood gas syringe into the baby — it contains a lot of heparin.
11 Slowly replace the fluid from the first 2 mL syringe.
12 Flush the line with heparinised Nsaline (2 units/mL); about 0.5 mL should suffice. Do it **slowly** at <5 mL/min

(i.e. 0.5 mL in >6 sec). Make sure this syringe is left empty on the 3-way tap after the procedure.

Clots which form on UA catheter tips actually form on damaged arterial intima, and this damage may be caused or accentuated by rapid fluid injection.

13 Before leaving the bedside, check that all arterial line connections are secure and open for infusion, and that blood isn't tracking back up the line.

Blood culture

The information obtained from a blood culture is extremely important for your assessment of a sick or potentially sick baby. It is, therefore, critical that the blood for culture be collected and handled in as sterile a fashion as possible.

- Best results are obtained by making the procedure for blood culture collection a separate procedure in its own right.

  It is usually 'false economy' to take a blood culture at the time of peripheral IV or IA insertion. Even taking blood from a cannula just after insertion has a significant risk of picking up skin organisms that are not true infecting organisms. Since skin organisms can be infecting organisms in premature infants, it is critical to exclude skin organism contamination from the blood culture bottle.
- Blood taken from an arterial line is acceptable for blood culture **only** when it is collected immediately after placement of an umbilical (not peripheral) line, while the operator is still 'scrubbed'.
- Blood may be taken by arterial or venous puncture, but the insertion site must not be touched after skin preparation.

Technique

1 Skin disinfection with an alcohol wipe, allowed to dry, is adequate.

2 After collection, a clean needle must be used to inject the blood into the blood culture bottle.

3 Aim to take 1 mL of blood. However, a smaller volume, if that is all that can be collected, may still be useful.

4 If blood for other tests is to be collected at the same time, the blood for culture must be placed into the blood culture bottle **before** attempting to transfer surplus blood to other sample containers for electrolytes, full blood count or other tests.
5 Send the blood culture bottle, properly labelled, to the bacteriology department as soon as practicable. Do not refrigerate.

Notes on blood culture

For a diagnosis of coagulase negative staphylococcal septicaemia to be sustained, we would usually require the following:

1 The infant is sick, consistent with septicaemia — e.g. apnoea, poor perfusion, lethargy, increased oxygen needs; and
2 Haematological indices consistent with infection; and
3 The organism is cultured from two separately collected blood specimens, or from two sites — such as the blood and a central catheter tip.

Lumbar puncture

> **!** **Contraindications:** cardio-respiratory compromise, low platelets, coagulation disorder.

1 Full sterile technique (sterile gown, gloves, mask). Skin preparation is with alcoholic chlorhexidine, allowed to dry.
2 Use a 22G lumbar puncture needle, in the L3–L4 space.
3 Have the nurse hold the baby with the spine flexed, and head extended (to avoid airway obstruction), positioned right on the edge of the mattress.
4 Insert needle about 0.5 (small preterm) to 1 cm (full term).
5 Collect at least 10 drops into each of 3 specimen containers.
6 Send the cerebrospinal fluid to microbiology as soon as possible for: microscopy and culture; protein; glucose;

and sometimes bacterial antigens, viral studies (polymerase chain reaction [PCR] and culture) or metabolic tests.

Bladder aspirate

This is best done when the infant's bladder is full. This will not always be known, so confirmation with ultrasound is useful.

1 Use a 23G needle with a 3 mL or 5 mL syringe.
2 Disinfect the skin with an alcohol wipe — allow to dry.
3 Insert the needle 0.5–1 cm above the symphysis pubis in the midline. The bladder is an abdominal organ in neonates.
4 Push the needle down perpendicular to the skin (i.e. angled a little towards the head) — about 1–2 cm is adequate.
5 Aspirate as you advance the needle until you hit the bladder (i.e. when urine is aspirated into the syringe).
6 Once urine is coming, fill the syringe, remove the needle, and place urine into a sterile container.

Endotracheal intubation

- For elective intubations, use a sterile intubation set.
- Try not to let the baby get cold.

Sedation

If the baby's condition requires urgent intubation, you should not wait for the sedation to be prepared for injection.

For non-urgent intubations, sedation (±analgesia ±paralysis) is desirable. This makes it easier on both the baby and the operator. Many different combinations are used. Common regimens are:

- morphine and midazolam — give a bolus of 50–100 μg/kg (i.e. 0.05–0.1 mg/kg) of each. [They can be given as a one-off injection, or as a bolus of 2.5–5 mL of the 'standard solution' (see page 83)]
- atropine 20 μg/kg, fentanyl 2 μg/kg, suxamethonium (i.e. succinylcholine) 1–3 mg/kg (given in that order)

- atropine 20 μg/kg, morphine 0.1 mg/kg, suxamethonium (i.e. succinylcholine) 1–3 mg/kg (given in that order).

What size endotracheal tube (ETT) to use?

This is not rocket science!

Gestational age	Size of ETT
<30 weeks	2.5 mm
30–35 weeks	3.0 mm
35–40 weeks	3.5 mm
>40 weeks	4.0 mm

Remember: 25–2.5; 30–3.0; 35–3.5; 40–4.0; or GA ÷ 10.

How far should the ETT go in?

This is not rocket science either!

- For oral endotracheal intubation use the 1 2 3 4 / 7 8 9 10 rule to gauge initial insertion — i.e. 1 kg = 7 cm at lip. See Figure 3.5.
- If using nasal tubes add 1 cm to the insertion distance.

Technique for endotracheal intubation

Make sure the baby is adequately oxygenated using bag-and-mask IPPV (intermittent positive-pressure ventilation) before each intubation attempt.

1. Cut the ETT to the desired length (insertion distance +4 cm) and insert the ETT connector and then the introducer. The introducer should be at the tip of the ETT but should not protrude beyond it.
   Some do not use an introducer at all; this will vary with operator preference.
2. If using a curved-blade laryngoscope, hold the tube in a sterile towel to bend the introducer through a smooth curve (that matches the curve of the laryngoscope blade), then make sure the introducer is able to be removed from the ETT easily. Don't handle the tube with your fingers.
3. View the larynx using the laryngoscope. Don't hyper-extend the neck. Use cricoid pressure.

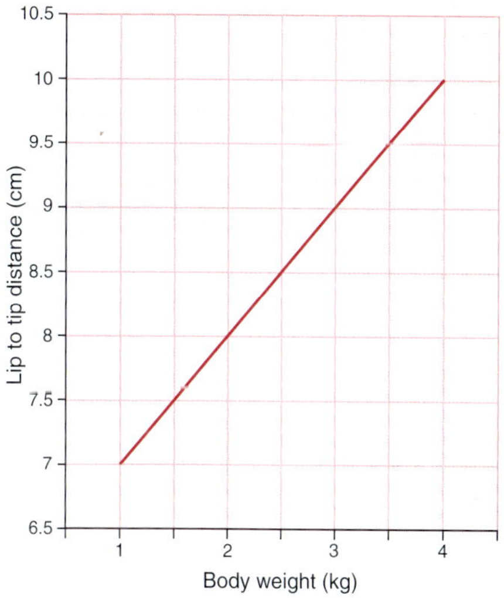

Figure 3.5 ETT insertion distance — oral insertion

4 Hold the ETT with its blue line facing you — i.e. the blue line on the ETT towards the nose or vertex of the baby.
5 Insert the ETT.
6 Limit each intubation attempt to under 30 sec.
7 After intubation, strap the ETT in place and obtain a chest X-ray to check its position. ETT tubes should always be strapped with the blue line (on Portex tubes) at the upper lip to ensure correct orientation of the bevel at the lower end.
8 X-rays should be taken with the head turned to the side, and should include the mouth end of the ETT to enable correct assessment of its placement.

The mid-point of the trachea is at T1. The carina is at T4. The ETT tip position should be mid-trachea, but is adequate if it is 1 cm above the carina (and no lower).

CHAPTER 4

Respiratory support

Mark Davies, David Cartwright and Luke Jardine

Respiratory distress

Respiratory distress, and the need for respiratory support, is one of the most common problems seen in neonatal units. Respiratory distress is **characterised** by one or more of the following:

- tachypnoea (>60 breaths/min)
- expiratory grunt
- recession (of any soft tissue around the thorax — e.g. intercostal)
- nasal flaring
- cyanosis.

The most common **cause** is hyaline membrane disease (HMD), also known as infant respiratory distress syndrome. The most important cause is infection (see pages 107–12).

Other causes soon after birth include: retained fetal lung fluid (also known as transient tachypnoea of the newborn or 'wet lung'); meconium aspiration syndrome; other aspiration syndromes (blood or liquor); air leak (pneumothorax or pulmonary interstitial emphysema); pulmonary hypoplasia (usually due to a space-occupying lesion in the chest, such as in congenital diaphragmatic hernia, or oligohydramnios); pleural fluid; and airway obstruction.

Other late-onset causes include: infection (viral or bacterial); chronic lung disease; chylothorax; and heart failure secondary to a left-to-right shunt.

The general **principles of management** include:

- put the baby somewhere you can watch it — admit to nursery

- monitor respirations, heart rate, oxygen saturation
- give just enough oxygen and no more (reasonable oxygen saturation targets are shown in the table on page 39)
- take a blood culture and start antibiotics
- give intravenous fluids
- chest X-ray (CXR) — exclude causes that may alter management, such as air leak, diaphragmatic hernia or pleural fluid
- consider respiratory support.

Continuous positive airway pressure (CPAP)

CPAP is a method of respiratory support used in the care of preterm and term infants. Indications for CPAP include:

- respiratory distress
- apnoea of prematurity
- airway obstruction
- post-extubation in very low birth weight infants.

Delivery methods vary according to institution, and include single prong (long or short), bi-nasal prongs (long or short), or mask.

The **aim of CPAP** is to hold the alveoli and airways open and prevent them collapsing during expiration. It therefore protects functional residual capacity, allowing the lungs to operate at maximal efficiency (by optimising their position on the pressure–volume curve). CPAP also stabilises the ribcage, reduces chest wall distortion during inspiration, and increases the efficiency of the diaphragm. It also regulates the respiratory rate (because of stimulation of the Hering–Breuer reflex) and results in increased inspiratory time and tidal volume. When given via the nose (nasal CPAP or NCPAP) it dilates the upper airway, which may explain its benefit in mixed or obstructive apnoea.

The **benefits of CPAP** include: a reduction in the need for intermittent positive-pressure ventilation (IPPV); decreased rate and severity of apnoea; increased chance of successful extubation; and decreased respiratory acidosis and oxygen requirements post-extubation.

The **risks of CPAP** include a potential for an increased incidence of intraventricular haemorrhage, nasal trauma and pneumothorax, as well as increased nursing care and the cost of consumables.

Starting CPAP: try a starting CPAP of 7 cmH_2O (range 5–10). This may be decreased or increased depending on the level of oxygenation and severity of apnoea.

Nasal intermittent positive-pressure ventilation (NIPPV)

NIPPV is a simple, effective mode of respiratory support where the infant is given CPAP plus a background ventilator rate with a set PIP (peak inspiratory pressure). A synchronised ventilator setting should be used.

It is more effective than CPAP alone in facilitating successful extubation and may also be useful in preventing intubation in apnoea of prematurity. Concerns have been expressed over a possible increased rate of gastrointestinal perforation, but this has not been supported in systematic reviews and may be minimised by using synchronised ventilation.

To place the infant on NIPPV:

1. Choose the ventilator mode of synchronised intermittent mandatory ventilation (SIMV).
2. Set the PEEP (positive end expiratory pressure).
3. Set the PIP (peak inspiratory pressure) — use a PIP 2–4 cmH_2O above that used pre-extubation, usually 14–20 cmH_2O.
4. Set the rate to 10 breaths per minute (range 10–25).

These settings may be increased or decreased depending on the level of patient oxygenation and severity of apnoea.

Surfactant

- Intra-tracheal surfactant is usually given to intubated infants with HMD — the earlier the better.

- Natural, animal-derived surfactants are usually used. We reccomend Survanta (Beractant, Abbott Pharmaceuticals) — the dose is 4 mL/kg, repeated if necessary after 6 hours.
  Other types are:
  - Curosurf (poractant alfa, Genepharm Pty Ltd) — 2.5 mL/kg
  - bLES (bovine Lipid Extract Surfactant, bLES Biochemicals, Inc.) — 5 mL/kg.
- Give surfactant by 2 hours if fraction of inspired oxygen $FiO_2 > 0.3$. Repeat at 6 hours if $FiO_2 > 0.25$.
- For babies <1250 g, give surfactant immediately if $FiO_2 > 0.3$ or PIP > 18 cmH_2O (before lines and X-ray).
- It is reasonable to give immediately to all babies <30 weeks gestational age who are intubated at birth.

Surfactant administration

It is not clear which is the best method of giving surfactant; there are variations in the methods of administration between and within different neonatal units. Administration of the total surfactant dose into four equally divided aliquots is the method recommended by the manufacturer of Survanta. Some administer it as a slow instillation via an endotracheal tube (ETT) over 5–10 minutes. However, animal studies have shown that a more rapid single bolus gives more uniform pulmonary distribution and dispersion of surfactant.

General

- With any of the methods below it will be necessary to recover or maintain chest movement with each mechanical ventilation breath by increasing the PIP.
- If oxygen saturation SpO_2 falls below 90%, increase the FiO_2 as well as increasing the PIP.
- If you do need to increase the PIP, make sure you turn it down again soon after: watch the chest wall movement. Volume-targeted ventilation is useful in this situation.
- Check an arterial blood gas within 30 minutes of giving surfactant.

Initial preparation

Position the baby supine and flat (i.e. without any rotation to either side) with the head in the midline. The ETT tip should ideally be in the mid-trachea. The surfactant should be at room temperature.

Method 1

- Use a 5FG infant feeding catheter cut to the length of the ETT and no longer.
- Disconnect the ventilator tubing manifold from the ETT connector.
- Place the cut feeding tube down the ETT. The tip should be at the tip of the ETT and not beyond.
- Instil the surfactant into the distal ETT over 10–20 seconds, then reconnect the manifold to continue IPPV.

Method 2

- Connect a blunt 18G drawing-up needle onto the syringe and instil the surfactant into the ETT connector via the suction port on the ventilator tubing manifold.
- Give over 2–5 minutes as tolerated. Continue mechanical ventilation throughout.

Method 3

- Instil surfactant via the side-port of an ETT connector over 2–5 minutes as tolerated.
- Continue mechanical ventilation throughout.

Assisted ventilation

The decision to ventilate a baby with respiratory distress needs to be taken in discussion with the relevant consultant. Generally accepted criteria are:

1 **Apnoea unresponsive** to stimulation or other treatment, OR:
   a **frequent**: more than 6 episodes in 6 hours requiring stimulation;
   b **severe**: more than 1 episode requiring bag-and-mask ventilation.

2 **Acidosis**, either:
  a **respiratory** acidosis: arterial pH <7.25 with a $PaCO_2$ (partial pressure of carbon dioxide in arterial blood) above 60 mmHg; or
  b **metabolic** acidosis: pH <7.25 or BE (base excess) worse than −10, not corrected by bicarbonate or volume loading.

3 Babies **requiring an FiO_2 >0.5** to maintain oxygen saturation >85%.

Babies <1500 g birth weight who need ventilation from delivery should remain ventilated until their respiratory status has fully declared itself.

> **!** Remember, respiration aims to:
> **get O_2 in** and **get CO_2 out**

- **To get O_2 in** all you need is a supply of inspired O_2 and:
  — expanded peripheral lung units (usually alveoli) that contain oxygen at a concentration higher than in the pulmonary capillaries, and
  — blood flow past those lung units — i.e. ventilation/perfusion (V/Q) matching.
- **To get CO_2 out** all you need is to wash CO_2 out of the peripheral lung units so that the concentration is below that in the pulmonary capillaries — i.e. ventilation or movement of gas in and out of the lung units.

Conventional mechanical ventilation (CMV)

- The basic form of IPPV or CMV used in neonates is pressure-controlled, time-cycled.
- Inspiration continues up to a maximum set pressure (peak inspiratory pressure, PIP) for the duration of the inspiratory time (IT).
- The length of expiratory time (ET) is either set on the ventilator or determined by setting IT and rate (breaths/min).

- During expiration the pressure is maintained at a set positive end expiratory pressure (PEEP).
- The pressure wave form, as measured at the proximal end of the ETT, is shown in Figure 4.1.

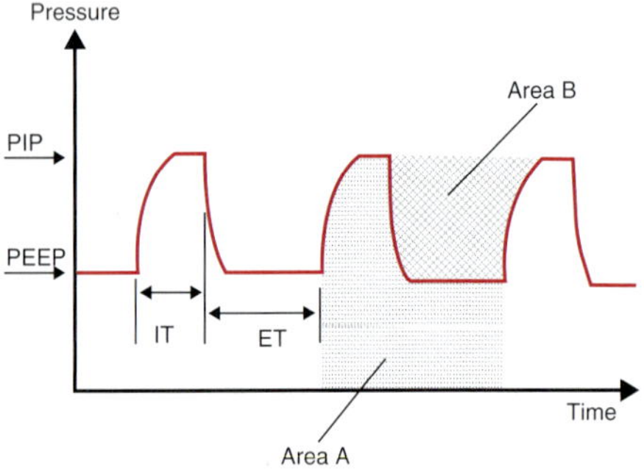

Figure 4.1 Pressure wave form for conventional mechanical ventilation (CMV)

ET = expiratory time; IT = inspiratory time; PIP = peak inspiratory pressure; PEEP = positive end expiratory pressure

To improve oxygenation (i.e. ↑ PaO_2):

— increase Area A and/or FiO_2

i.e. increase PIP, increase PEEP, increase IT, increase FiO_2.

To improve ventilation and CO_2 clearance (i.e. ↓ $PaCO_2$)

— increase Area B and/or rate

i.e. increase PIP, decrease PEEP, increase ET, increase rate.

Obviously, changing Area A will change Area B. A compromise needs to be reached.

In general: adjust pressure or rate to alter $PaCO_2$, and adjust FiO_2 to alter PaO_2.

Oxygen and CO_2 targets

Note: 1 kPa = 7.5 mmHg.

In general, it is not desirable to aim for normocarbia or normoxia. A $PaCO_2$ between 45 and 55 mmHg is acceptable. Oxygenation can be assessed by pulse oximetry, and if the baby requires oxygen then the following target ranges are reasonable.

Gestational age	SpO_2 target range
<30 weeks	85–92%
30+ weeks	90–94%

SpO_2 = oxygen saturation

Other settings

- An insipratory time (IT) of 0.5 seconds is adequate. Rarely would a longer IT be used.
  Some neonatologists use shorter ITs when ventilating babies with poorly compliant lungs.
- Adjust PIP to achieve adequate chest wall movement or a measured expired tidal volume (TV) of ~4 mL/kg (optimising minute ventilation if rate = 60).
- 4 mL/kg TV may be inadequate for extremely low birth weight infants (especially those <750 g). However, this is still a good starting point and further adjustments can be made titrated to $PaCO_2$.

Changes in respiratory status

Keep in mind the anticipated changes in the severity of the lung disease, and therefore changing compliance, of the lung. This will change depending on the natural course of the lung disease and any treatment given (e.g. lungs get better after surfactant and compliance improves). This will guide how often arterial blood gases (ABGs) need to be done.

- When lung disease and lung compliance are at their worst you need to adjust ventilation settings to achieve O_2 and CO_2 targets — i.e. tuning or fine-tuning IPPV.
- When lung disease is getting better you will be adjusting ventilation settings in response, usually by turning down PIP and/or rate — i.e. weaning.

- When lung disease is changing rapidly, especially if getting worse, ABGs may need to be done frequently, possibly every $^1/_2$ hour.

Always respond to changes in respiratory status by:

1. **examining the patient** (for chest wall movement, air entry, blocked tube or signs of a pneumothorax); and
2. considering checking ABGs and chest X-ray.

Such **changes in respiratory status** may include:

- significant change in FiO_2 (↓ / ↑)
- baby with increased spontaneous respiratory effort.

Significant **worsening ventilatory status** should prompt examination and investigation for:

- blocked or malpositioned ETT
- pulmonary air leak — pulmonary interstitial emphysema (PIE) or pneumothorax (PTX)
- atelectasis — generalised or focal.

Volume-targeted ventilation

Many ventilators now offer the option of volume-targeted ventilation. The ventilator will pick a PIP to use to target a set TV.

An example is the *Volume Guarantee* mode available on the Dräger Babylog 8000+ (Dräger Medical, Germany).

> *Volume Guarantee* is useful at times where there is rapidly changing compliance (e.g., after giving surfactant) or immediately after intubation when compliance is not known. It cannot be used when there is a large air leak around the ETT during inspiration (~>35%) or when the baby has significant spontaneous breathing.
>
> *Volume Guarantee* is not the same as 'volume-controlled' ventilation — *Volume Guarantee* is still pressure-controlled, but the ventilator is choosing which PIP to use breath-by-breath based on the 'target' tidal volumes you choose (i.e., the set TV).
>
> As a safeguard you still set an absolute maximum PIP that the ventilator will not exceed.

Volume-targeted ventilation is especially useful for small babies (<1250 g) who are more prone to the damaging effects of volutrauma and ventilator-induced lung injury.

Other similar, but by no means equivalent, types include: Targeted Tidal Volume mode on the SLE5000 (SLE systems, UK); and a number of different modes on the Stephanie paediatric ventilator (F. Stephan Biomedical, German), among others.

High-frequency ventilation (HFV)

CMV with large pressure gradients and large tidal volumes can cause ventilator-induced lung injury and its sequelae — worsening of acute lung disease, air leaks (pulmonary interstitial emphysema and pneumothorax) and chronic lung disease. To avoid these problems, the faster than normal respiratory rates used during HFV allow the use of small tidal volumes.

HFV **aims** to achieve adequate gas exchange (oxygenation and CO_2 removal) without the costs of barotrauma, atelectotrauma, and volutrauma.

HFV has two basic **components**:

1. A background continuous distending pressure (analogous to CPAP or PEEP), which is called the mean airway pressure (MAP). This produces continuous background inflation and recruitment of lung volume to achieve oxygenation.
2. 'Oscillation' of the airway pressure about the MAP at high frequencies. This is called the amplitude (or ΔP), and it determines the amount of alveolar ventilation and CO_2 removal (Fig 4.2).

Optimal HFV is achieved by producing and maintaining optimal lung expansion. This is often referred to as a 'high-volume strategy'. MAP is adjusted to optimise oxygenation. Increases in MAP lead to the recruitment of more alveoli and improved lung volume — this can be monitored by its effects on oxygenation, FiO_2 and CXRs. The aim is to achieve maximum alveolar recruitment without over-distending the lungs.

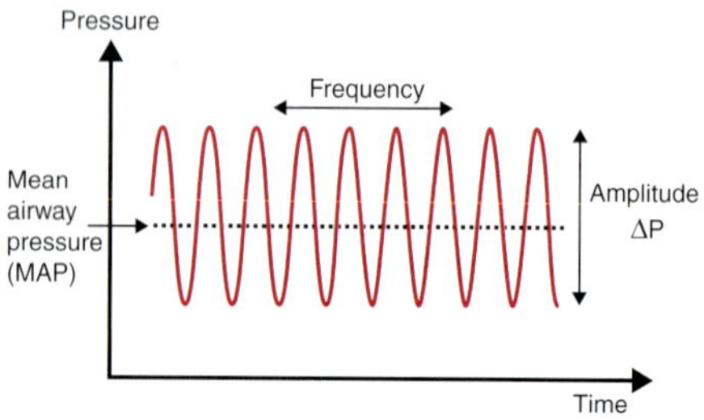

Figure 4.2 Pressure wave form for high-frequency ventilation (HFV)

Ventilation is optimised by adjusting **amplitude** (ΔP) to achieve a desired $PaCO_2$. The amplitude of each HFV 'breath' appears large compared with the PIPs used during CMV. However, the pressures are attenuated as they are transmitted down the ETT and airways so that the pressure oscillation is quite small at the lung periphery (Fig 4.3).

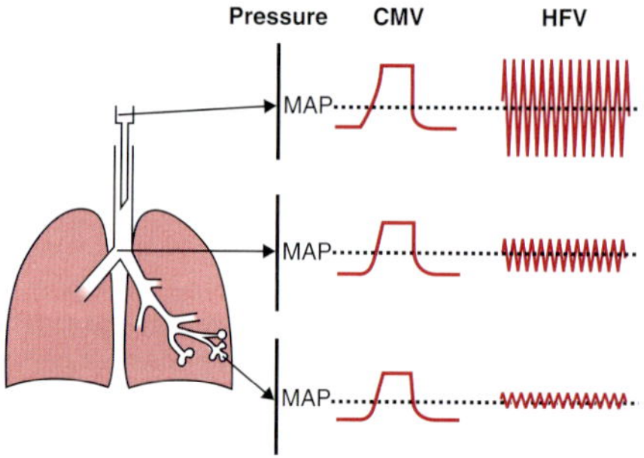

Figure 4.3 Attenuation of the HFV pressure wave form
CMV = conventional mechanical ventilation; HFV = high-frequency ventilation; MAP = mean airway pressure

Higher amplitude will increase tidal volume and improve CO_2 clearance (i.e. decrease $PaCO_2$).

As the ventilator **frequency** is increased, the lung impedance and airway resistance will increase and the tidal volumes decrease. Therefore increasing the frequency may decrease CO_2 clearance and increase $PaCO_2$. Conversely, decreasing the frequency often improves CO_2 clearance (although this will lead to less attenuation of the pressure oscillations and higher pressures transmitted to the alveoli).

Starting, changing and adjusting ventilation

Starting HFV

- A CXR before starting HFV is useful as a baseline measure of lung volume.
- Consider replacing the ETT with a larger one if there is significant leak around it.
- Where skin condition allows, transcutaneous O_2 and CO_2 monitoring should be commenced, as rapid changes can occur when changing to HFV, especially a rapid drop in $PaCO_2$.
- Oxygen saturation monitoring and an arterial line for ABGs and BP monitoring should already be established.
- Optimal pulmonary blood flow will require good blood pressure and perfusion. These should be optimised with volume replacement ±inotropes as necessary.
- Muscle relaxants are not indicated unless already in use.
- Sedation is used according to current unit policy.
- Low-compliance ventilator circuits are preferable.
- Use a low-volume humidifier chamber and keep it adequately filled — increasing compressible gas volume can affect amplitude.

Changing from CMV to HFV

- Leave the FiO_2 the same as on CMV.
- Set the frequency between 10 and 15 Hz (inclusive). The optimal frequency for HFV may be different in different disease states. Small infants with HMD may be

managed at higher frequencies, and term infants may be best managed at lower frequencies. With very non-compliant or stiff lungs, even lower frequencies may be necessary.

- Decrease the conventional breath rate and increase MAP simultaneously over 10–30 seconds until you reach the desired MAP. The desired MAP will usually be 2–4 cmH_2O above the MAP used when the infant was on CMV. MAP is regulated by using the CPAP or PEEP control on some ventilators.
- Set the amplitude (ΔP) until there is a discernible chest wiggle.
- A background conventional breath rate may be set on some ventilators — this is not essential when changing over to HFV and can be omitted.

Fine-tuning or weaning HFV

Oxygenation and ventilation are usually considered separately; however, changing one will often affect the other. **Always check all the settings** after making any adjustment.

Ventilation

To **change the $PaCO_2$** change the amplitude (or occasionally the frequency).

- To get rid of more CO_2 and therefore lower $PaCO_2$, ventilation may be increased by raising the amplitude.
- To decrease CO_2 removal and therefore increase $PaCO_2$, decrease the amplitude.

If adjustment of frequency is needed, decreasing the frequency increases CO_2 removal (the opposite to CMV). Always discuss this option with the consultant. (The response to a change in frequency may vary with different ventilators — the Infant Star has a fixed inspiratory time of 0.018 sec; the Dräger and SLE2000 have fixed I:E ratios so lowering the frequency will increase the IT.)

If there is still **poor CO_2 clearance** (i.e. high $PaCO_2$):

- Is the ETT blocked? Check for chest wiggle and breath sounds. Suck out or replace the ETT as necessary.

- Is there a pneumothorax? Transilluminate the chest, get a CXR.
- Increase the amplitude and see if the chest wiggle improves.
- Are the lungs under- or over-inflated? Get a CXR.
- If already at maximum amplitude, try reducing the frequency — lung impedance and airway resistance will fall, increasing tidal volume and CO_2 clearance.

Oxygenation

- Oxygenation is **controlled** by adjusting the MAP and FiO_2. The high-volume strategy dictates decreasing the FiO_2 first — therefore the MAP is usually not weaned until the FiO_2 is <0.4.
- The **degree of lung inflation** can be assessed by CXR. Arrange for a CXR when gases are stable to assess lung volume — usually 1–2 hours after starting HFV and every 12–24 hours after that.
- **Normal inflation** should allow the right hemi-diaphragm to be at about the 10th rib (posteriorly). Once the baby is stable in an FiO_2 <0.4, the MAP should be cautiously reduced by 1 cmH_2O as allowed by the oxygenation. If the FiO_2 rises, this suggests you have dropped MAP too much.

If **oxygenation remains poor** (i.e. low oxygen saturations or PaO_2):

- Is the ETT blocked? Check for chest wiggle and breath sounds. Suck out or replace the ETT as necessary.
- Is there a pneumothorax? Transilluminate the chest, get a CXR.
- Are the lungs not inflated enough? Try increasing the MAP, get a CXR.
- Are the lungs over-inflated? Check for hypotension. Try decreasing the MAP — does oxygenation improve? Get a CXR.

Over-distension of the lungs with a MAP that is too high can impede venous return and/or pulmonary blood flow. This will decrease systemic perfusion and worsen oxygenation. If the baby is hypotensive or has a metabolic acidosis, the lungs may be over-inflated. Get a CXR. Try decreasing the MAP — does oxygenation improve?

Trigger ventilation modes

Modern neonatal ventilators have many different modes of triggered ventilation available. The main aim of these modes of ventilation is to synchronise the baby's breath with that delivered by the ventilator. These modes rely on the baby's breath being detected by the ventilator in sufficient time to allow the ventilator to begin a mechanical breath while the baby is inspiring.

There are a few different types of triggered ventilation, and they are often called different names by different ventilator manufacturers. Common types are:

- **synchronised intermittent mandatory ventilation** (SIMV) — the ventilator delivers a mandatory number of breaths (set by the operator) at a set PIP and IT, but it will attempt to synchronise these mandatory breaths with the baby's inspiration.
  - If the baby is apnoeic, the ventilator will deliver the set rate of breaths at the set PIP and IT.
  - If the baby is spontaneously breathing, it will receive only the set number of mandatory ventilator breaths as well as its own spontaneous breaths.
- **synchronised intermittent positive-pressure ventilation** (SIPPV), also known as patient triggered ventilation (PTV) or assist control (A/C) — each spontaneous breath triggers a ventilator breath at a set PIP and IT.
  - If the baby is apnoeic, a back-up rate (set by the operator) will be delivered at the set PIP and IT.
  - If the baby is spontaneously breathing, it will receive a ventilator breath for each spontaneous breath (if breathing faster than the set back-up rate). If the baby breathes rapidly, you will need to decrease the IT.
- **pressure support ventilation** (PSV) — each spontaneous breath triggers a ventilator breath at a set PIP, but the IT is determined by the baby in that inspiration stops when the baby stops inspiring.

— If the baby is apnoeic, a back-up rate (set by the operator) will be delivered at the set PIP and a set IT.
— If the baby is spontaneously breathing, it will receive a ventilator breath for each spontaneous breath (if breathing faster than the set back-up rate).

Each of these modes can be combined with volume-targeted ventilation as described above.

Pneumothorax (PTX)

Needling the chest for a PTX

A procedure that is both diagnostic and therapeutic.

Site

Stay away from the heart, the internal mammary artery and the intercostal arteries — use either:

- 2nd intercostal space, mid-clavicular line — 2ICS, MCL; or
- 4th intercostal space, anterior axillary line — 4ICS, AAL.

Insert the needle as close as possible to the upper edge of the lower rib.

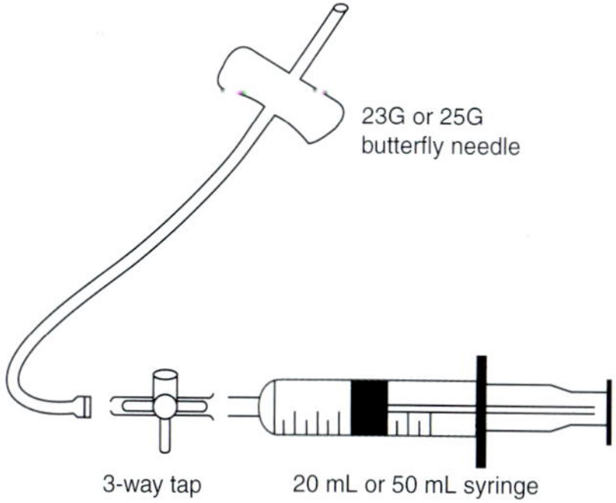

Figure 4.4 Equipment for 'needling' a PTX (pneumothorax)

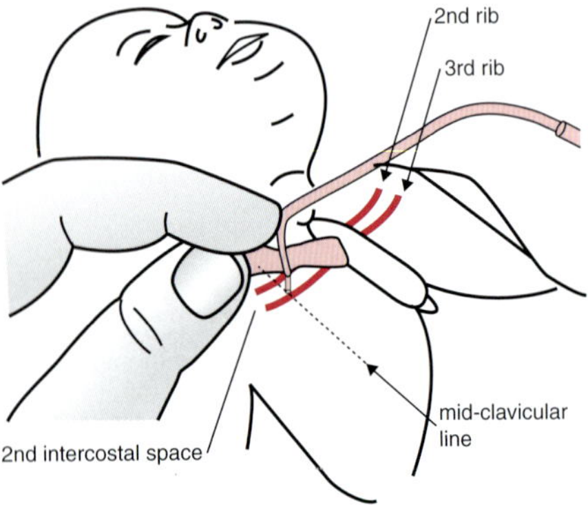

Figure 4.5 Site for 'needling' a PTX (pneumothorax)

Equipment

Attach a 23G or 25G butterfly needle to a 3-way tap attached to a 20 mL or 50 mL syringe. (See Fig 4.4.)

Procedure

1 Prepare the skin with an alcohol wipe and let dry.
2 Insert the needle perpendicular to the chest wall (straight down) $^1/_2$–1 cm in a small baby, 1–2 cm in a large baby.
3 Open the tap to the syringe and needle.
4 Aspirate — if the syringe fills with gas then there is a PTX. If you only get a few bubbles and some serous fluid it is not a PTX (yet!).
5 Open the syringe to the atmosphere (i.e. closed to the needle).
6 Empty syringe.
7 Repeat steps 3 to 6 until you are unable to aspirate any more gas. Note the amount of air aspirated from the pleural cavity (you can get up to 40–50 mL from a small baby and more than 200 mL in a large baby).
8 Remove needle — no dressing required.

Notes

- Be very careful that you do not empty the syringe back into the baby.
- If there is an ongoing air leak, you may need to leave the needle in situ and repeat the procedure until you can insert an intercostal catheter (ICC), especially if there is a tension PTX.
- After needling a chest for a PTX an ICC will usually need to be inserted.

Intercostal catheter (ICC) placement

> **!** The distance markings on the Argyle catheter are in centimetres from the most proximal side-hole, **not** from the tip. Insertion at the 1 to 2 cm mark is very adequate for a small baby, and at the 3 cm mark for a large baby.

General

- This is a sterile procedure.
- The best insertion site is in the mid to anterior axillary line, 5th–6th intercostal space, well away from the nipple.
- Use local anaesthetic if there is time.

Procedure

1. Make a deep hole down through the parietal pleura using first a No. 11 scalpel blade and then artery forceps. Once the hole is made you are ready to insert the catheter.
2. It is helpful to bend the trocar (1.5–2 cm from the tip) about 20–30° to aid in directing the ICC tip anteriorly.
3. Insert the catheter perpendicular to the skin. During insertion guide the tip of the catheter in the desired direction. This is facilitated by the bend in the catheter. **Never** use any force to insert the catheter through the chest wall.
4. The use of the trocar to puncture the hole through the pleura is **extremely** controversial. **Either:**

a the trocar is **never** used to make the hole between the skin and intra-pleural space, it is merely used to guide the direction of catheter placement (i.e. antero-inferiorly); i.e. the hole in the chest wall should be

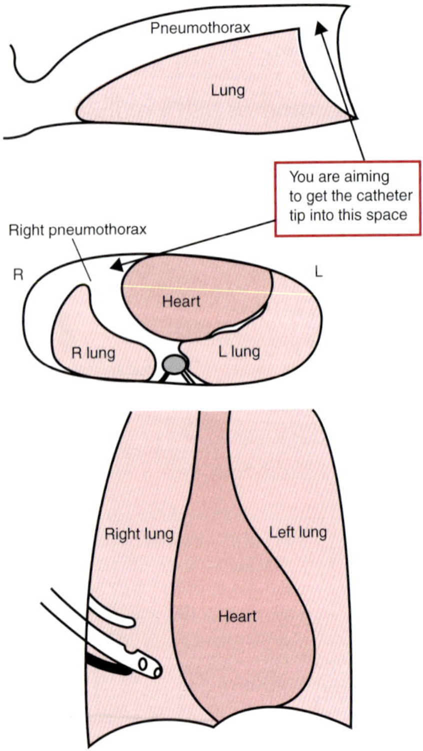

Figure 4.6 Correct position of tip of intercostal catheter (ICC)

complete before the catheter and trocar go anywhere near the baby; OR

b use the trocar to make the hole through the pleura, **but note** that this is only safe if it is held with both hands, using both index fingers ~1–1.5 cm from the tip, and all movement is from the elbows.

5 The ICC tip should be directed anteriorly (to lie in front of the lung), and infero-medially, towards the xiphisternum. It will then lie at the uppermost part of the pleural cavity when the patient is lying supine, i.e. at the antero-inferior rib margin. Free air will always rise and sit in the uppermost part of any cavity — this is where the catheter holes should be.

6 Always get a CXR after inserting an ICC.

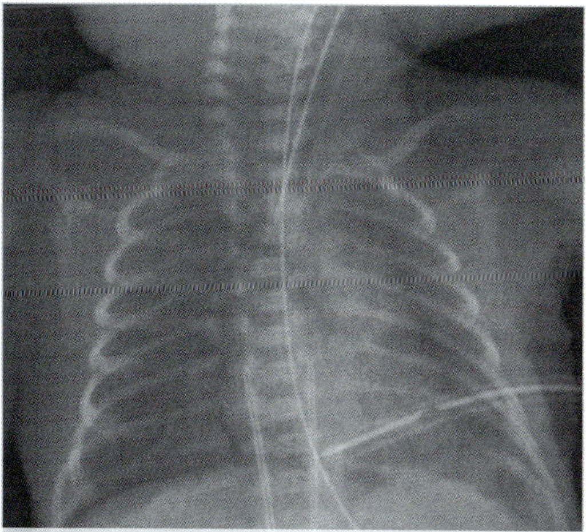

Figure 4.7 Chest X-ray of correctly positioned intercostal catheter (ICC) tip

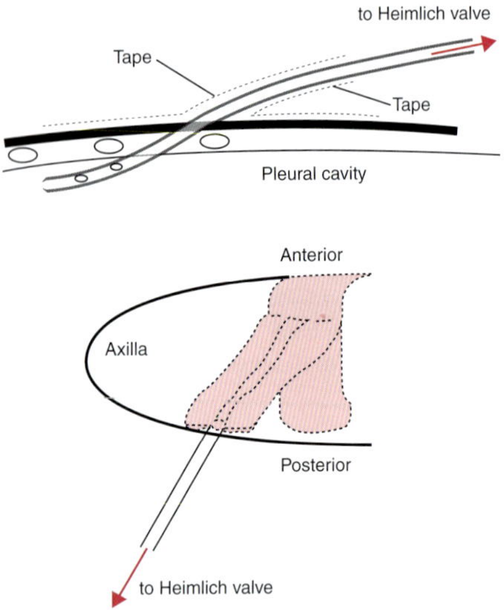

Figure 4.8 Taping in an intercostal catheter (ICC)

Notes

- It is normally not necessary to apply suction to an ICC. A Heimlich valve is quite adequate.
- Don't suture the ICC in place: this produces a puckered scar.
- Taping with a transparent, bio-occlusive, polyurethane dressing (such as Bioclusive, Tegaderm, Opsite) is adequate: sandwich the catheter between 2 pieces of dressing (Fig 4.8) — make sure the skin is dry.
- Make sure the catheter still points in the right direction — i.e. antero-infero-medially. To facilitate this, the external part of the ICC should be placed under the ipsilateral arm, running up past the head.

CHAPTER 5

Blood gas results

David Cartwright and Mark Davies

Blood gas report

Each intensive care unit should have an on-site blood gas machine. All give similar results.

The blood gas machine discussed here as an example is the Radiometer ABL 730. For blood gas analysis it measures three blood gas parameters — pH, PaO_2 and $PaCO_2$. A printed report from this machine is shown on page 54 as an example. Since, clearly, different machines will give different reports, it is important to be aware of exactly what your unit's machine measures and reports. The report in the example is divided into eight parts:

1 patient identification

2 blood gas values — the other values derived from these, in subsequent sections of the report, are either calculated or estimated. They have the subscript 'c' for calculated, or 'e' for estimated (for those involving the alveolar gas equation, which makes some assumptions)

3 blood oximetry values — displaying measured values for total haemoglobin (*c*tHb), oxygen saturation (sO_2), and proportions of some unusual haemoglobin compounds, such as fetal haemoglobin (HbF)

4 electrolyte values for Na^+, K^+, Cl^-, ionised Ca^{2+}

5 values for glucose, lactate, bilirubin

6 oxygen status

7 acid–base status calculations — actual base excess and actual bicarbonate (see below)

8 other calculated values — anion gap, $pO_2(A–a)_e$, $pO_2(a/A)_e$ (see below).

Figure 5.1 shows an example from the Intensive Care Nursery (ICN) gas machine at the Royal Brisbane and Women's Hospital.

RADIOMETER ABL 700 SERIES		
ABL RWH ICN	12:35:00	
PATIENT REPORT	Syringe - S 95uL	Sample #
Identifications		
Patient ID		
Patient first name		
Patient last name		
Operator		
Sample type	Arterial	
$FO_2(I)$	0.800	
PIP	21.0 cmH_2O	
PEEP	7.0 cmH_2O	
CPAP	14.0 cmH_2O	
Set RR	80.0 b/min	
Ti	0.4 seconds	
NO	15 ppm	
Blood gas values		
pH	7.375	
pCO_2	47.1	mmHg
pO_2	175	mmHg
Oximetry Values		
ctHb	147	g/L
sO_2	99.5	%
FO_2Hb	98.2	%
FCOHb	0.6	%
FmetHb	0.7	%
FHbF	81	%
FHHb	0.5	%
Electrolyte Values		
cNa^+	138	mmol/L
cK^+	4.7	mmol/L
cCl^-	102	mmol/L
cCa^{2+}	1.35	mmol/L
Metabolite Values		
cGlu	7.3	mmol/L
cLac	1.6	mmol/L
ctBil	143	μmol/L
Oxygen Status		
ctO_{2c}	20.6	Vol%
$P50_c$	21.80	mmHg
Acid Base Status		
ABE_c	1.6	mmol/L
$cHCO_3^-(P,st)_c$	25.8	mmol/L
Calculated Values		
Anion Gap_c	9.0	mmol/L
$pO_2(A\text{-}a)_e$	344.6	mmHg
$pO_2(a/A)_e$	33.7	%

Figure 5.1 Example blood gas result

Notes on calculated values

Standard bicarbonate, $cHCO_3^-(P,st)_c$

The standard bicarbonate is a notional value for the bicarbonate concentration that would be present in the sample of blood if the $PaCO_2$ were 40 mmHg. Its variance from a normal value of 24 indicates metabolic acidosis (<24) or metabolic alkalosis (>24).

We suggest using base excess (see below) rather than bicarbonate for these types of interpretations.

Actual bicarbonate

The actual bicarbonate is the bicarbonate content of the sample, calculated from the Henderson-Hasselbalch equation:

$$pH = pK + \log \frac{cHCO_3^-}{0.031 \times PaCO_2}$$

This value varies in proportion with changes in $PaCO_2$, in contrast with the standard bicarbonate which will not change with changes in $PaCO_2$, only with changes in acid or base content of the blood sample. Note in the examples below, all calculated on the same sample of blood, how the actual bicarbonate reflects the $PaCO_2$ changes, while the standard bicarbonate and base excess remain constant

Table 5.1 Example calculated values for actual bicarbonate (HCO_3^-)

pH	7.125	7.205	7.25	7.375	7.5
$PaCO_2$ (mmHg)	80	59	50	30	17
Actual HCO_3^-	26.3	23.3	21.8	17.5	13.2
Standard HCO_3^-	19.7	19.7	19.7	19.8	19.8
Base excess	–5.6	–5.8	–5.8	–5.8	–5.8

! Care must be taken to use the **standard** not the actual bicarbonate whenever you attempt to draw conclusions about a baby's acid–base status from the 'bicarbonate'.

Base excess

Base excess (BE) is the difference between the 'buffer base' of the measured sample and 'normal buffer base'. BE approximates the amount of acid or base needed to titrate 1 litre of blood to pH 7.4. 'Acidosis' and 'alkalosis', as we use the terms physiologically, are relative to a pH of 7.4. Blood with pH 7.4 and $PaCO_2$ 40 mmHg at 100% O_2 saturation has a base excess of zero (0.0). A negative BE (actually a base deficit) indicates metabolic acidosis; and a positive BE indicates a metabolic alkalosis. The BE, therefore, indicates the metabolic contribution to any measured acidosis or alkalosis.

For example, in the first example in Table 5.1 above, with a pH of 7.125, there is only a small metabolic acid contribution to this significant acidosis (BE –5.6). The major contributor to the acidosis is the high $PaCO_2$ of 80 mmHg (i.e. respiratory acidosis). A contrasting pH of 7.125 with a $PaCO_2$ of 40 mmHg has no respiratory contribution, and a major metabolic contribution with a BE of –16. A spontaneously breathing newborn baby with this degree of metabolic acidosis would more likely have a $PaCO_2$ of around 28 mmHg, created by over-breathing in response to the low pH — thus raising the pH to 7.19, a partial 'respiratory compensation' for a metabolic acidosis.

Note that the BE also can have a 'standard' and an 'actual' value, with different connotations from those of bicarbonate. The standard base excess (SBE) applies to the BE of the extracellular fluid, while the actual base excess (ABE) applies to that of the blood only.

Alveolar–arterial difference in partial pressure of oxygen, $pO_2(A–a)_e$

This is derived from the alveolar gas equation. A large pO_2(A–a) value indicates that there is a lot more oxygen in the alveolus than in the arteries, and the patient has a serious problem getting oxygen into the blood from the alveoli. There is a major ventilation–perfusion (V/Q) mismatch and/or a major gas diffusion problem.

Arterial/alveolar ratio of partial pressures of oxygen, $pO_2(a/A)_e$ (a/A ratio)

This is simply another way of expressing the difference between alveolar (A) and arterial (a) pO_2, by expressing one as a fraction of the other. Here it is printed as a percentage, but may also often be quoted as a decimal fraction (e.g. 0.337 equates to 33.7%).

In clinical studies examining the effectiveness of Exosurf (a synthetic surfactant), an a/A ratio of ≤0.22 was the most commonly used index of severity of disease. An a/A ratio of 0.22 approximates having a PaO_2 of 50 mmHg in 50% oxygen, with a reasonably normal $PaCO_2$.

Partial pressures of oxygen at 50% saturation, $p50(act)_c$ and $p50(st)_c$

The pO_2 values at 50% saturation for your actual sample (act) and your sample without fetal haemoglobin (st) tell you whether the patient's oxygen–haemoglobin dissociation curve is 'left-shifted'.

Blood oximetry values

These are *measured* values. The haemoglobin (Hb) is measured, and the oxygen saturation is assessed using the absorbance at multiple wavelengths of light. The co-oximeter in the blood gas machine needs to make a correction to its measured values because of its use of multiple wavelengths of light. The machine uses its calculated fetal haemoglobin (HbF) concentration for this correction.

The pulse oximeters we use to monitor babies do not need correction of their values for HbF concentration (hence their usefulness), because they measure at only two wavelengths (660 and 940 nm) where the differences in absorption between fetal and adult haemoglobin of the same saturation are insignificant.

Many preterm infants have a HbF concentration in excess of 90% at birth. Term infants have about 80%. The cHbF drops quickly with transfusion, which is always with adult blood.

Alkalosis

In neonatal practice two causes of metabolic alkalosis are seen:

1 chronic diuretic administration, with hypochloraemia; and
2 compensation for chronic respiratory acidosis.

In the latter, the patient does not actually become 'alkalaemic'. An example would be pH 7.35, $PaCO_2$ 80 mmHg — the BE would then be +14.5.

Acidosis

In neonatal practice, many instances of respiratory and metabolic acidosis are seen. In treating these, the best principle is to treat respiratory acidosis with respiratory treatments, and treat metabolic acidosis with metabolic management (e.g. administration of alkali, volume expansion for better perfusion). Many times it is appropriate to accept a respiratory acidosis, particularly in an infant with respiratory disease who is spontaneously breathing. Treatment of respiratory acidosis in a ventilated infant will depend on the underlying lung pathology. The principle is to increase alveolar ventilation. See section on conventional mechanical ventilation, page 37.

Treatment of metabolic acidosis with $NaHCO_3$ is most efficient in the absence of a concomitant respiratory acidosis, since the reaction

$$HCO_3^- + H^+ \longleftrightarrow H_2CO_3 \longleftrightarrow H_2O + CO_2$$

must occur for the bicarbonate to 'mop up' hydrogen ions. If CO_2 cannot be removed there is little point in administering bicarbonate, e.g. if the $PaCO_2$ is >60 mmHg.

- When bicarbonate is given, it should be given slowly, at a rate not exceeding 1 mmol/min (i.e. 1 mL/min of 8.4% $NaHCO_3$).
- No dose should be given over less than 5 minutes.
- Be sure that all bicarbonate has cleared the line before sampling for further blood gas analysis if giving through a UAC (umbilical arterial catheter).

- Never give bicarbonate in the same line as calcium — it makes concrete!

> A 'half-correction' dose of sodium bicarbonate $NaHCO_3$ to give for metabolic acidaemia can be calculated from:
>
> Dose in mmol $NaHCO_3$ =
>
> $$\frac{\text{Weight in kg}}{4} \times \text{Actual base excess}$$

- Two sources of spurious metabolic acidosis sometimes occur when blood gases are measured — contamination of the sample with 10% dextrose, and contamination of the sample with heparin. These can be avoided by correctly preparing syringes for the latter, and correctly following line sampling procedure for the former (see pages 25–6).

CHAPTER 6

Pulmonary hypertension

Mark Davies

Description

Whilst pulmonary artery pressures are increased in this condition, the main pathophysiological problem is the restriction of pulmonary blood flow due to increased pulmonary vascular resistance.

Some degree of pulmonary hypertension will be present with any significant lung disease (such as hyaline membrane disease, HMD); we usually use the term when there is significant pulmonary blood flow restriction and hypoxia due to:

1 pulmonary hypoplasia (e.g. diaphragmatic hernia, oligohydramnios)
2 increased pulmonary arteriolar muscle constriction (which may be sensitive to hypoxaemia and acidaemia)
   — primary (i.e. no apparent cause) — once known as persistent fetal circulation
   — secondary to lung disease, such as meconium aspiration syndrome or infection.

Management

- Cover for bacterial infection — give antibiotics.
- Sedation.
- Hyper-oxygenation, paralysis and forced alkalosis are no longer routinely recommended.
- Optimise lung volume. Lung disease and ventilation-perfusion (V/Q) mismatch are important — get the lungs expanded first.

- Optimise circulation — correct any hypovolaemia, use inotropes.
- Pulmonary vasodilation — nitric oxide (NO) is the best agent (see below).
- With ventilation:
    - make sure you have adequate PEEP (positive end expiratory pressure)
    - aim for pre-ductal oxygen saturation SpO_2 of 90–94%
    - $PaCO_2$ of 45–55 mmHg is adequate ($PaCO_2$ = partial pressure of carbon dioxide in arterial blood)
    - high-frequency ventilation (HFV) may be needed to achieve adequate lung expansion.
- Confirm raised pulmonary artery pressures with echocardiography — this will also exclude congenital cyanotic heart disease.

Some neonatologists still chase hyperoxia and aim for SpO_2 (pre- or post-ductal) of 99–100% or high PaO_2 values.

Inhaled nitric oxide (iNO)

- Nitric oxide (NO) is a potent vasodilator and it can be added to the inspiratory line of the ventilator. Thus the NO in the inspired gases will get to the pulmonary arterioles and dilate them.
- It has an ultrashort half-life, so it does not get into the systemic circulation.
- There is a theoretical risk of platelet dysfunction, and you must monitor for methaemoglobinaemia (metHb is available on some gas machines; >5% is bad).
- **Dose:** use 10–20 ppm.
- Wean slowly when able, e.g. when FiO_2 is <0.4.
- Inhaled NO will be next to useless if there is significant atelectasis, V/Q mismatch and/or poor circulation.

CHAPTER 7

Patent ductus arteriosus (PDA)

Garry Inglis

Features

The ductus arteriosus usually closes functionally by 48 hours and anatomically by 3 weeks of age in well, term babies. Closure may take longer in preterm or unwell babies.

PDA is associated with increased risk of death, intraventricular haemorrhage (IVH), chronic lung disease, necrotising enterocolitis and impaired renal function; although a causal relationship has not been proved. Most PDAs are asymptomatic and there is no uniformity in the approach to management of PDA. Many will eventually close spontaneously without any specific intervention. Only a small number will cause heart failure. Complications of PDA are related, at least theoretically, to shunting through the duct, circulatory overload and the 'diastolic steal' phenomenon.

Ductal reopening after closure is uncommon.

Diagnosis

The diagnosis of PDA is best done using echocardiography. Clinical signs of a PDA often lag behind the echocardiographic findings by several days, consistent with findings that clinical diagnosis has very low sensitivity. The specificity of many clinical features is also low, as is the inter-observer agreement of the presence of signs. Classical signs that may be sought include:

- systolic or continuous murmur

- wide pulse pressure and bounding pulses
- active precordium
- hepatomegaly
- chest X-ray changes — increased heart size, increased vascularity.

A chest X-ray has been found to add very little to the other clinical signs in the diagnosis of PDA. In high-risk babies, most but certainly not all systolic murmurs will indicate the presence of a duct. Remember also that some babies (including preterm ones) will have a duct-dependent cardiac lesion.

Decision to treat

The decision to treat a PDA should be based on more than just finding it. Factors such as the baby's age and gestational age, general condition, and degree of left-to-right shunting should be taken into account. Systematic reviews have not shown any significant benefit to treatment of asymptomatic nor symptomatic PDA. However, most neonatologists would have difficulty ignoring a symptomatic duct and many also choose to treat asymptomatic ducts under some circumstances.

Information that may be provided by the cardiologist or echocardiographer that would indicate a more significant or 'troublesome' duct includes:

- size of the duct
- direction of the shunt
- dilatation of the left heart — a left atrial : aortic root ratio >1.48 is significant
- absent or reversed diastolic flow in the descending aorta.

An assessment of left ventricle function (usually the fractional shortening) is also useful.

Treatment options

Treatment options include cyclo-oxygenase inhibitors or surgical ligation — this is discussed further below.

Indomethacin

Reasonably strong evidence is available to support the use of prophylactic indomethacin, where those at high risk of PDA are given treatment early — usually within 12 hours of birth. This has been shown to be quite safe and significantly reduces the incidence of PDA, the need for medical or surgical treatment of PDA, and grade 3 or 4 IVH.

As there are no proven long-term benefits (e.g. survival, neurosensory impairment), some neonatologists choose not to use prophylaxis.

- Treatment or prophylaxis usually consists of intravenous indomethacin (see page 81 for regimens). It should be given by infusion over at least 20 minutes.
- Enteral indomethacin should be avoided if possible.
- Contraindications to the use of indomethacin include duct-dependent congenital heart disease, significant renal disease, oliguria (<0.5 mL/kg/hr over 24 hours has been used in some trials), platelet count $<50 \times 10^9$/L, overt bleeding (other than pulmonary haemorrhage).
- Side effects include decreased urine output, oedema, hyponatraemia and gastrointestinal bleeding.
- Some use ibuprofen instead of indomethacin.

Fluid restriction

There is some evidence to suggest that babies managed with more restricted fluid intake in the first several days of life have lower risk of PDA than those whose fluid intake is more liberal.

Our preferred approach to fluid administration is regarded as being on the 'restrictive' end of the spectrum. This should be distinguished from fluid restriction as an approach to the management of PDA. In the presence of a large shunt and heart failure, it is sensible to use fluid restriction with or without diuretics. With asymptomatic or uncomplicated PDA, however, it is illogical to fluid-restrict, and doing so by 20–30 mL/kg/day (as is frequently done) probably achieves nothing other than denying important calories to the baby.

Surgical ligation

There is no good evidence to support the use of duct ligation as initial management of PDA under normal circumstances. Likewise, it is not clear whether those whose medical treatment has failed to close the duct benefit from ligation.

Ligation can be achieved via a number of approaches, which will be surgeon-dependent. Most babies who undergo ligation have a left lateral thoracotomy and the duct is either sutured or clipped.

Post-operative morbidity can include vocal cord paralysis, chylothorax, pneumothorax, exacerbation of chronic lung disease, thoracic scoliosis, infection and significant pain. Accidental ligation of the left pulmonary artery or aorta has been reported.

CHAPTER 8

Thermoregulation

David Cartwright

Background

- Temperature regulation is critical to survival of preterm babies. They have few mechanisms for losing heat if too warm, a high surface-area-to-volume ratio making heat loss easy, and few mechanisms for increasing body temperature when cool.
- Preterm babies have much lower body fat stores than term babies, particularly of 'brown fat' which is a good energy store that is able to be converted to heat readily.
- Very preterm babies have very thin, permeable skin, which allows increased water loss across the skin. This evaporative water loss is also a potent source of heat loss. Some units use a plastic wrap to ameliorate this heat loss before admission to the nursery.
- It is best to avoid hyperthermia.

While there are good data showing that the long-term management of preterm babies in suboptimal environmental temperatures is associated with poorer survival, and there are data showing an association between low admission body temperature and poorer survival, there are no data which show that admission hypothermia and the subsequent short-term hypothermia that occurs in the intensive care unit are causative of that poorer outcome. Admission hypothermia could simply be a marker for sicker infants who have already required more than usual intervention and who will have poorer outcomes. It cannot be assumed that making babies warmer at admission will improve their survival — more research is needed to determine a causal link between transient hypothermia and poor outcome, and whether improving admission temperatures is an effective intervention.

Techniques

The 'thermo-neutral range' for environmental temperature (i.e. the environmental temperature at which a baby's energy expenditure is lowest) is generally higher and narrower the more immature the baby. We need to provide warmth and minimise radiant and evaporative heat losses.

1 Provide warmth — generally an incubator or open bed with radiant warmer is used.
   We recommend using incubators exclusively for all preterm babies; be aware of the slightly increased difficulty in performing vascular access procedures that comes with that. These procedures really can be performed very readily inside incubators, particularly the more modern, roomier ones. Some units, however, prefer to initially nurse a baby under a radiant warmer. The use of radiant warmers increases evaporative fluid losses.
2 Minimise radiant heat losses — have the room in which the babies are kept warmed to 24–26°C. A double-walled incubator also assists in reducing radiant heat losses.
3 Minimise evaporative heat losses — use an incubator rather than an open bed with a radiant warmer. Provide high humidity — many of the newer incubators can do this very efficiently. Use as much humidity as is possible while avoiding 'rainout' in the incubator — in the order of 60–80%.
4 The heat outputs of both incubators and radiant warmers can be servo-controlled to the baby's skin temperature, which is a more sensitive indicator of a cool infant than its core temperature. A baby in a suboptimal thermal environment will maintain its core temperature longer than its skin temperature, but this will be at the expense of energy that should be used for breathing and growing. Skin servo-control can be a very efficient method of allowing the baby to determine its own neutral thermal environment: set the skin temperature 0.5–1°C below core temperature, e.g. 36.2–36.5°C.

CHAPTER 9

Blood pressure

Mark Davies

Reference values

Some reference values for blood pressure are given below. **These values are a guide only.** The adequacy of an individual infant's blood pressure (BP) and the possible need for treatment should be based on clinical factors (e.g. peripheral perfusion, urine output, BP waveform, metabolic acidosis) in addition to these values.

Mean arterial blood pressure

Table 9.1 Lower 95% CI for mean arterial blood pressure (mmHg) in VLBW infants

Time since birth	Gestational age (weeks)									
	23	**24**	**25**	**26**	**27**	**28**	**29**	**30**	**31**	**32**
0–12 hrs	20	21	22	23	25	26	27	28	29	30
13–24 hrs	20	22	23	25	27	28	29	30	32	33

[Data from: Lee J, Rajadurai VS, Tan KW. Blood pressure standards for very low birthweight infants during the first day of life. Arch Dis Child Fetal Neonatal Ed 1999;81(3):F168–F170.]

CI = confidence interval; VLBW = very low birth weight

Systolic blood pressure

Table 9.2 Systolic BP (mmHg): age 4–24 hours

	Gestational age (weeks)				
	24	**28**	**32**	**36**	**40**
97th percentile	57	62	67	74	82
3rd percentile	27	29	33	36	40

See Table 9.3 for older infants

Table 9.3 Systolic BP (mmHg): age 10 days

	Gestational age (weeks)				
	24	**28**	**32**	**36**	**40**
97th percentile	71	84	94	104	111
3rd percentile	34	40	45	50	54

[Data in Tables 9.2 and 9.3 (approximate values from graph) from: Anonymous. Systolic blood pressure in babies of less than 32 weeks gestation in the first year of life. Northern Neonatal Nursing Initiative. Arch Dis Child Fetal Neonatal Ed 1999;80(1):F38–F42.]

Treatment options

Low BP in a newborn infant may be due to a number of factors including hypovolaemia, myocardial insufficiency, low peripheral vascular resistance, patent ductus arteriosus or any combination of these.

- If hypovolaemia is suspected it is reasonable to give 1–2 doses of 10 mL/kg Nsaline (Normal saline, 0.9%); or in some units colloid, e.g. albumin.
  - If there is no response after 2 doses of plasma expanders then inotropes are usually considered as the next option (unless the baby is still considered to be hypovolaemic).
  - Use dobutamine if myocardial insufficiency is suspected, and dopamine if low peripheral vascular resistance is suspected.
- Recalcitrant hypotension can be treated with steroids:
  - hydrocortisone IV: 2.5 mg/kg 4 hourly initially; or
  - dexamethasone IV: 0.25 mg/kg.

CHAPTER 10

Fluids and nutrition

Mark Davies, David Cartwright and Garry Inglis

Renal function

There is a lot we do not understand about newborn renal function. Adult reference ranges of electrolytes etc may not be applicable to newborns, especially those who are preterm. **At birth**, serum electrolyte and creatinine values are usually similar to those of the mother.

It is normal for newborns to take up to 24 hours to **first pass urine** and they often have a urine output of <1 mL/kg/hr during the first couple of days. This period of relative oliguria is usually followed by a diuresis.

Average **glomerular filtration rate** is lower in newborns than in adults but serum creatinine levels tend to be lower also. Glomerular filtration rate may be influenced by factors such as medications (e.g. dopamine, indomethacin), hypoxic-ischaemic injury, a patent ductus arteriosus and respiratory distress.

Insensible **water losses** are proportionally greater in newborns than in adults. However, newborns are generally quite capable of maintaining adequate water balance over a wide range of fluid intake.

In practical terms, renal function and fluid balance can be **monitored** using serial weight measurements, urine output and serum sodium as guides. Serum potassium is often falsely elevated in newborns because of the method of collection (heel-prick collection causes haemolysis and/or contamination with tissue fluids). Serum urea and creatinine may be confusing and probably do not add a great deal to what can be determined by using the measurements noted above.

Parenteral fluids

General

- The standard parenteral fluid used initially in infants is 10% dextrose. This gives some caloric intake for those babies not fed for some time. Alternatively, a variety of starting fluids that may contain maintenance saline or calcium can be used.
- If given through an umbilical arterial line, heparin at a concentration of 1 unit/mL is added (500 units per 500 mL bag).
- Standard starting infusion rate is 60 mL/kg/day. For very small, preterm babies, 80–100 mL/kg/day may be started. This can then be varied according to serial weight measurements or electrolyte concentrations. **The initial infusion rate does not need to be routinely increased during the first three days of life, especially in infants with lung disease.**
- Do not increase fluids just because the urine output is poor. If the baby is not passing urine and the fluids are increased, you may cause fluid overload and hyponatraemia.

Electrolytes

- No standard electrolyte additives are normally necessary in the first few days. All preterm infants have an excess of extracellular fluid at birth and must undergo some electrolyte losses via urine when getting rid of this excess fluid.
- The most common fluid balance problem in the first 48 hours of life is excessive evaporative fluid loss in very small infants. This is reflected in excessive weight loss and rising serum concentrations of sodium and chloride ions, $[Na^+]$ and $[Cl^-]$. Electrolytes may need to be measured every 8 to 12 hours in extremely low birth weight (ELBW) infants in the first 48 hours, and fluid intake adjusted accordingly. Fluids do not need to be increased until the serum $[Na^+]$ is in the high 140s (in mmol/L).

- When Na^+ is added, the most convenient way to do so is to make a mixture in the burette of 80 mL 10% dextrose and 20 mL Nsaline (this is 8% dextrose/one-fifth Nsaline; Nsaline is Normal saline, 0.9%).
  Some units use a ready-made 10% dextrose/one-fifth Nsaline solution, and others add NaCl to a bag of dextrose. **Do not use** 20% SALINE in IV fluids except under exceptional circumstances. (20% SALINE contains 3.42 mmol/mL of Na^+ if you need it.)
- The addition of potassium K^+ should be undertaken with great caution. If required, it should be added to a burette, with the amount ordered in mmol **and** in mL to avoid confusion [e.g. 10% dextrose, 98 mL; KCl, 2 mL (= 2 mmol); run at 7 mL/hr]. It is safest for all burette additives to be ordered **in mL** of a stated concentration of the additive.

Other

- In most preterm infants the serum calcium concentration [Ca^{2+}] will decrease in the first few days, and the total serum [Ca^{2+}] will commonly be 1.5 mmol/L or less. There is good evidence that the ionised [Ca^{2+}] remains normal down to a total [Ca^{2+}] of 1.3 mmol/L.
- If hypocalcaemia is to be treated, the standard parenteral dose is 3 mL of 10% calcium gluconate/kg/day. Be very wary about giving this via a peripheral IV line, as nasty extravasation burns with necrosis occur if the line infiltrates. It is satisfactory to give this as an infusion into an umbilical artery, but boluses should be given very slowly and carefully.
- **Never** give Ca^{2+} into a peripheral arterial line. **Never** give calcium in the same line as bicarbonate or parenteral nutrition.
- Peripheral arterial line fluid is normally $^1/_2$N or Nsaline, given at 0.5–2 mL/hr. It should contain 2 units/mL of heparin. Such an infusion is best administered by syringe pump. **No drugs are ever administered via a peripheral arterial line.**

Parenteral nutrition (PN)

The provision of parenteral nutrition varies considerably from unit to unit. This variation is in: the solutions used and their composition; how the solutions are delivered; and when they are started and stopped.

- Parenteral nutrition usually consists of the infusion of a solution of amino acids (such as Vamin or Primene) and carbohydrate (dextrose), plus a solution of fat (Intralipid). Vitamins are also given, both water-soluble and fat-soluble.
- Some neonatal units make up individual prescriptions for PN with varying concentrations of dextrose and electrolytes on a base amino-acid solution. In practice this process is unwieldy and unnecessary. The baby is much smarter than you are at sorting out minor electrolyte problems.

A suggested procedure

- Use standard solutions with set concentrations of amino acids, dextrose, Na, K, Ca, Mg, Cl, P, Zn and Cu:
  - Our starting solution (Solution 1) has 1% amino acids and 10% dextrose plus electrolytes and trace elements.
  - Solution 2 has higher concentrations of amino acids (1.75%) and dextrose (12.5%).
- Start with Solution 1, at the same rate as the baby's maintenance fluids were being given, increasing by 20 mL/kg/day daily if fluid balance permits.
- Change the PN to Solution 2 after a couple of days (at the next line change). Total fluids are then usually increased (again if fluid balance permits) daily by 20 mL/kg/day up to 180 mL/kg/day. If the dextrose is not tolerated, insulin at 0.05–0.2 units/kg/hr can be infused — see page 83.
- Add water-soluble vitamins (e.g. Soluvit N) to the burette at the beginning of the first infusion after each line change (3 days per week — M,W,F), 2 mL/kg each time. The vitamins are thus given to the baby over the first few hours — minimising the vitamins' exposure to light.

- Give lipid as a 20% solution of Intralipid at a dose of 2 g/kg/day (10 mL/kg/day). Fat-soluble vitamins can be added as Vitalipid N — 4 mL/kg/day to a maximum of 10 mL/day. Other neonatal units will start at 1 g/kg/day and increase over a few days up to as high as 3 g/kg/day, with monitoring of triglyceride levels. Some stop lipid infusion if the baby has septicaemia; we don't.

General

- Parenteral nutrition should be administered via a central line or umbilical venous line.
- Parenteral nutrition given via peripheral lines must be very carefully managed as extravasation burns occur at sites of infiltration, and evidence from randomised controlled trials demonstrates that where peripheral IV lines are used the babies get much less nutrition because of the time spent without IV access.
- PN solutions and infusion lines are changed every 2–3 days. **Remember, all central line changes must be done as full sterile procedures.**

Enteral feeding

> **!** Feeding of breast milk is encouraged for all babies. Don't automatically stop breast milk feeds if the mother is on medications. Get advice from pharmacy or a Drug Information Centre first.

Preterm babies have four main difficulties with respect to feeding:

1. weak and incoordinated deglutition <34 weeks gestational age
2. small initial gastric capacity of ~3 mL/kg
3. poor gastrointestinal activity
4. poor digestive capacity (rarely of practical consequence).

Feeding therefore presents the need for:

1. intragastric tube feeding for babies <34 weeks gestational age

2. small initial feeds of 3 mL/kg usually
3. adequate spacing between feeds for gastric emptying — we use 3 hours to start with
4. graded increases in volume and frequency as tolerated.

If a baby is not being enterally fed, always ask yourself why not?

Babies who might not be started on enteral feeds from soon after birth include:

- ELBW babies
- babies who were growth-restricted in utero and who had absent/reverse diastolic flow in the umbilical artery
- babies with gut obstruction
- babies with significant respiratory distress
- those whose mothers wish to exclusively breast feed but have not produced any expressed breast milk (EBM) yet.

Feeding regimes

- In a well baby, who is able to tolerate full enteral feeds from day 1, feeds can be started at 60 mL/kg/day and increased to 180 mL/kg/day by day 7.
- A baby that is not fed and who is only getting a dextrose/saline solution (i.e. no feeds or PN) doesn't need more than 120–140 mL/kg/day of total fluids.

> Standard feeds contain 67 Cal/100 mL.
> Low birth weight (LBW) infant formulas contain 81 Cal/100 mL.

There are many ways to start small feeds and build them up slowly: from continuous to every 1, 2, 3 or 6 hours! Here is one scheme:

- Start all feeds as bolus feeds given every 3 hours, usually at around 2–3 mL/kg.
  - For babies weighing <1500 g, the aim is to change to feeds every 2 hours once tolerance of reasonable volumes 3-hourly has been established.
  - For babies weighing <1000 g, feeds can be increased by 1 mL per feed every 24 hours until 5 mL every

3 hours is reached. Then change to 4 mL every 2 hours, and increase by 1 or 2 mL every 12 to 24 hours as tolerated. Very rarely, hourly bolus or continuous feeds need to be given.
  - For babies weighing 1000–1500 g, the increases can be of larger volumes each feed, and undertaken every 12 to 24 hours.
- Feeds are usually changed back to being given every 3 hours when the baby's weight reaches 1600 g and if the feeds are well tolerated.

Supplementation of breast milk

Babies of <1500 g who are fed breast milk need supplementation with phosphate (to prevent osteopaenia of prematurity) and iron (to aid recovery from anaemia of prematurity). A baby's iron stores run out when it reaches twice its birth weight.

- For **phosphate,** either:
  - use Sandoz Phosphate tablet; dissolve 1 tablet into 16 mL of water (gives ~1 mmol/mL). Give 1 mL/kg/day of this mixture in 4 divided doses; this will give 1 mmol/kg/day of PO_4^{3-}; or
  - fortify feeds — use EBM with fortifier or an LBW formula.
- For **iron**, use iron solution, such as Fergon; give 2–6 mg/kg/day from 14 days of age, usually given twice a day (we recommend 0.5 mL twice a day).

Infants weighing <1500 g may benefit from 'fortification' of breast milk with a breast milk fortifier such as FM85 or Wyeth Breast Milk Fortifier. These fortifiers add protein, some starch calories, phosphate and calcium.

We do not recommend fortifying until feeds are well tolerated at good volumes. For artificially fed infants a LBW infant formula may be used. If the 'ready-to-feed' preparation is used, iron content is 8 mg/L (most normal, non-fortified baby formulas have 8–12 mg/L) and iron supplementation is not needed. Fortification is normally ceased when the baby weighs 2000–2500 g.

CHAPTER 11

Hypoglycaemia

Mark Davies and David Cartwright

Background

Hypoglycaemia is defined as a blood sugar level (BSL) of <2.6 mmol/L as measured by a bedside glucometer or a blood gas machine. 1 mmol/L = 18 mg/dL.

Blood glucose assessments should be routinely undertaken on premature infants, infants whose birth weight is <10th percentile for their gestational age, infants of diabetic mothers, and other macrosomic babies — at 1 hour, 2 hours and 4 hours of age, then every 4 hours for 24 hours until stable.

- The laboratory blood glucose is often higher than the bedside measurement.
- Any low or borderline BSL should be confirmed with a laboratory or a blood gas machine measurement.

Management

The basic principle of managing hypoglycaemia is to give the baby more sugar than it is currently getting.

Options for treatment are:

If BSL is 2.0–2.5 mmol/L:

1 Feed with milk (not glucose water).

2 Feed more frequently, e.g. every 1–2 hours if necessary.

If BSL is <2.0 mmol/L:

3 Start 10% glucose IV at 60 to 75 mL/kg/day.

4 Increase the dextrose infusion rate or concentration.

- Usually just increasing the amount of dextrose infused is enough — i.e either:
  - — increase the **rate** of infusion (e.g. from 0 to 60 mL/kg/day, or from 60 to 80); or

— increase the **strength** of the infusion (e.g. from 10% to 12% dextrose, then 14%, 18%). If you need to give more than 12% dextrose, use a central line or umbilical venous line.

> To make a solution of dextrose stronger than 10%:
> $^1/_{10}$ of the volume of 10% dextrose
> + $^1/_2$ of the volume of 50% dextrose
> = the % dextrose per 100 mL of solution.
> e.g. 95 mL of 10% dextrose + 5 mL of 50% dextrose
> = 9.5 + 2.5 = 12
> i.e. 100 mL of 12% dextrose.

Notes on dextrose

- Bolus doses of dextrose are almost never required and run the risk of rebound hypoglycaemia. **Rarely** a bolus may be needed: 2–3 mL/kg of 10% dextrose (200–300 mg/kg) initially.
- **Never** give a bolus of dextrose without increasing the amount infused as well.
- Check the BSL again 1 hour after any increase or bolus.

Additional drug treatment

Drug treatment may sometimes be necessary for hypoglycaemia that is not responding to simple measures as above. Next options for recalcitrant hypoglycaemia are to add hydrocortisone, glucagon, diazoxide or octreotide.

- **Glucagon** mobilises glycogen stores, so is not particularly useful for growth-restricted babies; it is good for infants of diabetic mothers and for other hyperinsulinaemic states.
  — The dose is 0.04 mg/kg IV or IM, then 10–50 μg/kg/hr. (1 mg/kg of glucagon made up to 50 mL in Nsaline gives a solution which when run at 0.5 mL/hr delivers 10 μg/kg/hr of glucagon. Nsaline is Normal saline, 0.9%)
- **Hydrocortisone** primarily increases gluconeogenesis and has a slow response.
  — The dose is 1 mg/kg/dose every 6 hours IV.

- **Diazoxide** and **octreotide** should be reserved for established diagnosis of hyperinsulinaemia, and used only after endocrinologist consultation.

Further investigation

An infusion of 60 mL/kg/day of 10% dextrose is approximately 4 mg/kg/min of dextrose. Infusion rates of >10 mg/kg/min (150 mL/kg/day) with persisting hypoglycaemia should be regarded with some suspicion, and may be indicative of hyperinsulinism. Under these circumstances, investigations (**at the time of hypoglycaemia**) should include:

- **Blood** – glucose, insulin (±C-peptide), cortisol, pH, lactate, ketones, growth hormone, adrenocorticotrophic hormone (ACTH), acylcarnitine profile.
  This can be achieved by collecting the following amounts of blood in the tubes indicated. The colours of blood specimen tubes will vary from hospital to hospital — always check.

Specimen type	Tube colour
3 mL clotted blood	red top
1 mL EDTA	pink top
2 mL heparin	green top

  Also collect an ABG (arterial blood gas) in a blood gas syringe and spots of blood on a standard neonatal screening card. If you can, always collect a little extra for each type of tube.
- **Urine** — amino and organic acids — collect the first urine passed after the episode of hypoglycaemia. The urine should be sent fresh to the lab immediately after collection. **Do not freeze.**

One should always keep inborn errors of metabolism in mind because many infants present with hypoglycaemia with or without metabolic acidosis, ketosis, hyper-ammonaemia, hyperuricaemia, etc. Other investigations might include a serum amino acid profile, ammonia, free fatty acids and pyruvate.

CHAPTER 12

Common drugs and infusions

Mark Davies and David Cartwright

Common drug doses

- Aminophylline (IV) or theophylline (oral/NG)
  - — loading…5 mg/kg
  - — maintenance…2 mg/kg/dose…every 8 hours
- Ampicillin (IV)…50 mg/kg/dose…every 12 hours
- Caffeine citrate (IV/oral/NG)
  - — loading…20 mg/kg
  - — maintenance…5–10 mg/kg/dose…daily
- Cefotaxime (IV)…50 mg/kg/dose…every 12 hours
- Chloral hydrate (oral/NG)
  - — hypnotic…50 mg/kg/dose…STAT
  - — sedation…6 mg/kg/dose…every 6 hours
- Dexamethasone…see pages 86–8
- Iron (oral/NG)…see page 76
- Flucloxacillin (IV)…50 mg/kg/dose
  - — first week of life…every 12 hours
  - — 2–4 weeks old…every 8 hours
  - — >4 weeks old…every 6 hours
- Frusemide (IV/oral/NG)…1–2 mg/kg/dose…every 12 hours
- Gentamicin (IV)…2.5 mg/kg/dose
  - — <30 weeks…every 36 hours
  - — ≥30 weeks…daily
  - — trough level, prior to third dose, <2 mg/L is OK

- Hydrocortisone (IV)…1–2.5 mg/kg…every 4–6 hours initially
- Indomethacin (IV) — a number of regimens exist:
  - — prophylaxis…0.1 mg/kg/dose…daily for 3 days
  - — treatment #1 (usual)…0.1 mg/kg/dose…daily for 6 days
  - — treatment #2…0.2 mg/kg/dose…every 12 hours for 3 doses
  - — treatment #3…0.2 mg/kg STAT…then 2 doses of 0.1 mg/kg…every 12 hours
  - — treatment #4…0.2 mg/kg/dose every 12 hours for 3 doses…then 0.1 mg/kg/dose daily for 4 or 5 days
- Midazolam (IV)…50–100 μg/kg/dose (i.e. 0.05–0.1 mg/kg)
- Morphine (IV)…50–100 μg/kg/dose (i.e. 0.05–0.1 mg/kg)
- Penicillin (IV)…60 mg/kg/dose… every 12 hours
- Phenobarbitone (IV/oral/NG)
  - — loading…20–30 mg/kg/dose
  - — further bolus…10 mg/kg/dose
  - — maintenance…2.5 mg/kg/dose…every 12 hours
- Phosphate (NG)…see page 76
- Ranitidine (oral/NG)…3–6 mg/kg/dose…every 8 hours
- Spironolactone (oral/NG)…1–2 mg/kg/dose…every 12 hours
- Theophylline see aminophylline
- Vancomycin (IV)…15 mg/kg/dose
  - — <1200 g…every 24 hours
  - — ≤7 days old, ≥1200 g…every 12 hours
  - — >7 days old, 1200–2000 g…every 12 hours
  - — >7 days old, >2000 g…every 8 hours
  - — (trough level, prior to third dose, 10–15 mg/L is OK)

Standard infusions

Note: Nsaline is Normal saline, 0.9%.

Dopamine

A powerful vasopressor agent used for elevating blood pressure (BP). At low doses it also increases urine output in adults. The 'renal dose' for neonates is not well documented, but is probably somewhat lower than that usually quoted for adults (0.5–2 μg/kg/min in neonates vs 3–5 μg/kg/min in adults). Dopamine stimulates dopamine receptors, is an alpha and beta agonist, and a serotonin agonist with varying effects at different doses.

Dose of dopamine

- Doses are:
  - For 'renal' purposes usually use 4 μg/kg/min, or less.
  - For BP, start at 10 μg/kg/min, but may be effective at 5 μg/kg/min, particularly in very immature infants.
- For both purposes, **mix in** Nsaline, 5% or 10% dextrose in a 'low-stiction' syringe, e.g. Braun or IVAC: **30 mg/kg of dopamine in 50 mL of fluid.** This gives a solution of dopamine 600 μg/kg/mL. **If run at 1 mL/hr, this is 10 μg/kg/min.**

  This may be doubled in strength if fluid management is a problem.
- Dopamine may be given in parenteral nutrition lines, before the filter. **Never** give into any arterial line.
- Dopamine is usually given via a peripheral venous line or a central venous line (CVL). It needs to be a line that is not having bolus drugs given through it. It is compatible with morphine/midazolam solution, and with parenteral nutrition solutions.

Dobutamine

An agent used to improve myocardial contractility (heart rate and strength of contraction — a beta agonist). Also has some pulmonary vasodilating effects, at least theoretically. Not as good as dopamine for elevating blood pressure, unless the cause of low BP is poor myocardial performance.

Dose of dobutamine

- Usually start at 10 μg/kg/min.
- **Mix in** Nsaline, 5% or 10% dextrose, in a 'low-stiction' syringe, e.g. Braun or IVAC: **30 mg/kg of dobutamine in 50 mL of fluid.** This gives a solution of dobutamine 600 μg/kg/mL. **If run at 1 mL/hr, this is 10 μg/kg/min.**
- May be given in parenteral nutrition lines, before the filter. **Never** give into any arterial line.

Insulin

For control of hyperglycaemia (sometimes seen in infants on IV dextrose, parenteral nutrition or dexamethasone).

Dose of insulin

- 0.05–0.2 units/kg/hr.
- **Mix in** Nsaline: **25 units/kg insulin in 50 mL of Nsaline. If run at 0.1 mL/hr, this is 0.05 units/kg/hr.**

Midazolam

Used for sedation or for seizures. Use with caution in unintubated, non-ventilated infants.

Dose of midazolam

- Infusion: the standard infusion rate is 6–10 μg/kg/hr (0.3–0.5 mL/hr).
- Single dose: for elective intubation, a bolus of 50–100 μg/kg (0.05–0.1 mg/kg) should be given prior to intubation.

  This can be given as a one-off injection, or as a bolus of 2.5–5 mL of the standard solution below (if the baby's clinical status can tolerate that much fluid), or intranasally (at double the dose).
- For both infusion and single dose, **mix in** Nsaline, 5% or 10% dextrose: **1 mg/kg in 50 mL of fluid**. This solution contains 20 μg/kg/mL.

  If run at 1 mL/hr, this is 20 μg/kg/hr.

Morphine

Used for sedation and/or pain relief — for ventilated infants only. Do not give to unintubated infants.

Dose of morphine

- Infusion: the standard infusion rate is 6–10 μg/kg/hr (0.3–0.5 mL/hr).
- Single dose: for elective intubation, a bolus of 50–100 μg/kg (0.05–0.1 mg/kg) should be given prior to intubation. Give as a one-off injection, or as a bolus of 2.5–5 mL of the standard solution below (if the baby's clinical status can tolerate that much fluid). (It is safer to give as standard solution to avoid accidental overdose.)
- For both infusion and single dose, **mix in** Nsaline, 5% or 10% dextrose: **1 mg/kg in 50 mL of fluid**. This solution contains 20 μg/kg/mL.

  If run at 1 mL/hr, this is 20 μg/kg/hr.

> Morphine and midazolam can both be put in the same syringe. 1 mL/hr gives 20 μg/kg/hr of each drug.

Prostaglandin — PGE_1

PGE_1 (Alprostadil) is used to open, or maintain open, the ductus arteriosus. It is a generalised vasodilator and has also been used in the management of pulmonary hypertension (with bigger doses).

Dose of PGE_1

- The usual starting dose is 0.005 μg/kg/min.
- **Mix in** Nsaline: **30 μg/kg in 50 mL of Nsaline**. **If run at 1 mL/hr, this is 0.01 μg/kg/min.**

  Therefore the starting infusion rate is 0.5 mL/hr.
- The solution may be made stronger (e.g. double concentration) for very small babies, to reduce the total amount of fluids given.

Beware of apnoea as a side effect. During retrievals ventilate the baby in case apnoea occurs in transit. Fever and flushing of the skin also occur. The fever is presumed to be a central effect.

CHAPTER 13

Chronic lung disease (CLD)

Mark Davies and Garry Inglis

Background

There is no uniform definition of chronic lung disease (CLD), or bronchopulmonary dysplasia (BPD). Definitions are usually based on the need for respiratory support (whether oxygen or mechanical support) at a specified time point (28 days of age and/or 36 weeks post-menstrual age is frequently used). The Australian and New Zealand Neonatal Network (ANZNN) defines it as 'any form of respiratory support (supplemental oxygen and/or assisted ventilation) for the initial chronic respiratory disease at 36 weeks post-menstrual age, in babies born at less than 32 weeks gestation'.

- Babies born at 23 weeks gestation have greater than 80% chance of getting CLD, decreasing to less than 10% in babies born at 31 weeks gestation.
- Babies with CLD have significant morbidity and it is a leading cause of late mortality.

Before discharge, babies with CLD require a longer duration of respiratory support (mechanical ventilation and continuous positive airway pressure) and oxygen treatment, and spend longer in hospital.

After discharge, many will need home oxygen and the rate of re-hospitalisation is high. Lung function measurements (especially measurements of air flow) are often below average, recurrent respiratory infections are common, and there is an increased risk of neurodevelopmental delay.

Management

The clinical course in babies with CLD will improve with time and growth — if they survive the respiratory failure that CLD brings. Numerous treatments have been tried to ameliorate established CLD. The mainstay of treatment remains postnatal systemic corticosteroids (see *Dexamethasone* below), but this has become increasingly controversial in recent years.

Other treatments that have been tried include inhaled steroids, bronchodilators, diuretics, fluid restriction, vitamin A, inhaled nitric oxide, sildenafil and erythromycin.

- Oxygen is given to target oxygen saturations >90% and <95%. Targeting higher saturations has been proven to be of no benefit and can become an endless cycle of increasing oxygen delivery.
- Some are aggressive in treating a patent ductus arteriosus in babies with CLD.
- Nutritional management is important — most of these babies need higher caloric intake than babies at similar ages without CLD.
- Some would consider respiratory syncytial virus (RSV) immunoprophylaxis.

Dexamethasone

For chronic lung disease (CLD)

Dexamethasone may be used for management of CLD, especially as an aid to weaning from assisted ventilation. Its use is controversial given an increased incidence of cerebral palsy (or an abnormal neurological examination), seen when multiple randomised controlled trials are combined in meta-analysis. However, it should be noted that the majority of trials allowed the use of dexamethasone in the non-treatment groups and the same meta-analysis showed no increase in the rate of disability.

- Dexamethasone is usually commenced at 7–14 days of age if ventilatory requirements are still significant, but is often started later than this.
- We suggest writing up the entire duration of the dexamethasone course at the beginning. This ensures that doses of dexamethasone are not overlooked during the course.

> **!** Be wary of infection when starting dexamethasone. In some smaller babies antibiotics may be used to 'cover' known colonising organisms over the first 4–5 days of a course.

Regimens

Numerous regimens for a weaning course of dexamethasone in CLD exist. Dexamethasone can be given intravenously (IV) or enterally.

Dexamethasone, 6-week course

- 0.5 mg/kg/day (given in two divided doses) for 3 days.
- Then 0.3 mg/kg/day (given in two divided doses) for 3 days.
- Then reduce dose by 10% each 3 days, until 0.1 mg/kg/day.
- Then 0.1 mg/kg/day (given in two divided doses) every other day for 6 days, and then cease.

[Avery GB et al. Controlled trial of dexamethasone in respirator-dependent infants with bronchopulmonary dysplasia. Pediatrics 1985;75:106–111.]

Dexamethasone, '2-week' course

- 0.5 mg/kg/day (given in two divided doses) for 3 days.
- Then 0.3 mg/kg/day (given in two divided doses) for 3 days.
- Then 0.2 mg/kg/day (given in two divided doses) for 3 days.
- Then 0.1 mg/kg daily for 3 days, and then cease.

Dexamethasone, DART protocol

- 0.15 mg/kg/day (given in two divided doses) for 3 days.
- 0.1 mg/kg/day (given in two divided doses) for 3 days.
- 0.05 mg/kg/day (given in two divided doses) for 2 days.
- 0.02 mg/kg/day (given in two divided doses) for 2 days.

[Doyle LW et al. Low-dose dexamethasone facilitates extubation among chronically ventilator-dependent infants: a multicenter, international, randomized, controlled trial. Pediatrics 2006;117:75–83.]

For airway oedema

Dexamethasone is sometimes given to prevent failure of extubation where there is suspected oedema of the vocal cords or sub-glottis. The course is:

- 0.25 mg/kg/dose every 8 hours for 3 doses, the last dose given 1 hour before extubation.

CHAPTER 14

Care of the extremely preterm baby

Mark Davies and David Cartwright

Initial care of the ELBW infant prior to transfer to Level 3 nursery

> Avoid birth outside a hospital with a Level 3 neonatal unit! Transfer in utero if possible.

Resuscitation

- A B C (airway, breathing, circulation).
- Intubate or not? This depends on the paediatrician's comfort zone — the default option is intubate and ventilate.
- Ventilation — beware high pressures, use peak inspiratory pressures (PIPs) just high enough to move the chest. Provide positive end expiratory pressure (PEEP) of 6–7 cmH_2O.
- Oxygen saturation — aim for 85–92%.

Intubation/Ventilation

- The only absolute indication is apnoea.
- This depends on the paediatrician's comfort zone — safest to intubate and ventilate unless baby looks very good.
- Endotracheal tube (ETT) size:
  - — use 2.5 if <1000 g
  - — try 3.0 if >1000 g.

- For oral ETT, tape at upper lip at:
  - 7.0 cm if ~1000 g
  - 6.5 cm if ~750 g
  - 6.0 cm if ~500 g.
- Chest X-ray — ETT tip should be at T1; should be at least 1 cm above carina (which is at T4).
- The enemy is atelectasis — use adequate PEEP: start with 6–7 cmH_2O.
- If on CPAP (continuous positive airway pressure), start with 7–8 cmH_2O; unless in air, then use 5 or 6 cmH_2O.
- Surfactant: unless in air on lowish pressures, give surfactant (Survanta 4 mL/kg; Curosurf 2.5 mL/kg).
- Ventilator settings — a good starting point is:
  - rate 60
  - inspiratory time 0.5 s
  - pressures (PIP/PEEP) 18/6 cmH_2O.

Adjust PIP according to chest movement or blood gas results; wean PIP until chest movement OK, then wean rate.

Oxygenation

- Saturations 85–92% — **never over 95%**. Don't chase after elusive high saturations.
- If oxygenation poor despite adequate $PaCO_2$ (partial pressure of carbon dioxide in arterial blood), then try:
  - increase PEEP
  - support heart: dobutamine, adrenaline
  - increase blood pressure (BP): dopamine, adrenaline.

  Always discuss inotrope use with a neonatologist before using.

Ventilation

- $PaCO_2$ — high 40s (mmHg) or low 50s is OK; don't chase normocarbia.
- Avoid $PaCO_2$ <30 mmHg (strong association with adverse neuro-developmental outcome and chronic lung disease).

- Sedation — morphine/midazolam if baby resists ventilation:
  - — bolus of 0.06–0.1 mg/kg each is usually enough
  - — can infuse at 10 μg/kg/hr each if needed
  - — see pages 83–4.

Antibiotics

- Just give them! Penicillin and gentamicin unless mother has other known bacteria — take blood culture first. (Green liquor — ampicillin instead of penicillin.)

Blood pressure

- MABP in mmHg > GA in weeks is OK — if well perfused. (MABP = mean arterial blood pressure; GA = gestational age.)
- Low BP: 10 mL/kg Nsaline (some use albumin) ×2, then dopamine 3–5 μg/kg/min (see page 82). Timing of second Nsaline/albumin dose depends on response to first. (Nsaline = Normal saline, 0.9%.)
- If evidence of acute blood loss — replace with blood.
- Inotropes — dobutamine, dopamine, adrenaline (discuss with a neonatologist).
- Steroids (hydrocortisone IV — 1–2.5 mg/kg every 4–6 hours).

Correct acidosis

- Give slow bicarbonate infusion (over longer than 5 minutes):
  - — Dose (in mL of 8.4% solution) =

$$\frac{\text{Birth weight (in kg)}}{4} \times \text{Base excess}$$

  or just give 1–2 mL/kg.

Vitamin K

- Smaller dose — 0.5 mg (i.e. 0.05 mL of Konakion MM Paediatric).

Fluids

- 80 mL/kg/day of 10% dextrose.

Thermoregulation

- Dry the baby immediately after birth or use a polyethylene wrap.
- Keep warm — skin temperature 36.3–36.8°C, axillary temperature 37°C.
- Woolly hat on baby, plastic or bubble wrap over baby, warmed humidified air into cot.
- If under a radiant warmer on an open cot, ensure skin temperature probe is covered with a reflective disc. **Do not** cover baby with blanket — that will stop the overhead warmer from warming the baby.

Lines

- Consultants only — put in an umbilical venous catheter (UVC) and maybe an umbilical arterial catheter (UAC). **Never use the second umbilical artery if unsuccessful with the first — leave that for the staff at the Level 3 neonatal unit.** An ELBW infant without adequate umbilical lines can be a major problem.
- Prep with **aqueous** chlorhexidine **only**.
- Measure tip of right shoulder to umbilicus — put UAC in this distance, or use the 'ready reckoner' tables on pages 166–8.
- Measure bottom end of sternum to umbilicus — put UVC in this far, or use the 'ready reckoner' tables on pages 166–8. UVC tip should be at the bottom of the heart between T8 and T9; if below T9 but good blood flowback when aspirated, then leave in place and use for 10% dextrose and urgent drugs.
- Do not use UVC for inotropes (or parenteral nutrition) unless tip is in the inferior vena cava or right atrium.

Skin

- No unnecessary tape.

Photographs

- … of the baby for parents to keep.

Mother

- Transfer to same hospital as baby as soon as possible, express breast milk.
- Warn parents — long time in hospital, intensive care nursery, on respiratory support and oxygen; neuro-sensory deficits; cerebral palsy; neuro-developmental problems; disability.

Guidelines for care of infants <1000 g / <28 weeks at a Level 3 nursery

1. Consultant or 'attending' neonatologist (and at least one registrar/fellow/resident/neonatal nurse practitioner) to be present at delivery.
2. Where indicated, intubate with a size 2.5 endotracheal tube (ETT) to:
   — 7.0 cm if ~1000 g
   — 6.5 cm if ~750 g
   — 6 cm if ~500 g.
   Use a Neopuff or similar T-piece device (see page 8) to deliver PEEP and ventilate to transfer to nursery.
   If not needing intubation, commence CPAP from delivery (Neopuff).
3. If ventilated:
   — ventilate in intensive care at 80/min, inspiratory time 0.38 sec
   — use volume-targeted ventilation (e.g. the Dräger ventilator with Volume Guarantee) 4 mL/kg
   — monitor oxygen saturation continuously; target 85–92%.
4. Do not use a transcutaneous blood gas monitor.
5. Superficial swabs (groin and ear).

6 Surfactant — give early rather than late:
- give to all babies in this group who need intubation at birth, as soon as the ETT is in place
- give immediately if fraction of inspired oxygen FiO_2 >0.3 or PIP >18 cmH_2O (before lines and X-ray)
- give by 2 hours and repeat 6 hours later (see page 35) if FiO_2 >0.25.

7 Insert:
- umbilical arterial catheter (UAC), 3.5FG — consultant or 'attending' neonatologist or a senior trainee should do this; little babies are not for learners.

  Check with consultant whether high (T8–T12) or low (tip below L2). Some recommend low, reasoning that the catheter is larger than 1/2 the diameter of the aorta so why potentially compromise gut and kidney blood flow with that above mesenteric vessels?
- umbilical venous catheter (UVC), double lumen 3.5FG; prime with heparinised Nsaline. (Nsaline = Normal saline, 0.9%.)

Run:
- UAC: Nsaline or 1/2Nsaline with 1 unit heparin/mL, 0.5 mL/hr
- UVC primary lumen: 10% dextrose to total fluids 60–80 mL/kg/day
- UVC secondary lumen: Nsaline (no heparin), 0.2 mL/hr.

> **!**
>
> Use great care in swabbing the abdomen.
> - Alcoholic chlorhexidine burns — apply very sparingly, with only a corner of the swab wet. **Never** allow **any** to run down the side of the abdomen.
> - It's the alcohol that burns — **never** allow a baby to lie in this. **Never** apply any dressing over wet alcohol.
> - We recommend aqueous chlorhexidine — it's easier and safer, especially in an emergency situation.

8 Antibiotics — penicillin 60 mg/kg every 12 hours and gentamicin 2.5 mg/kg every 36 hours.

9 If platelet count is >50 × 10^9/L then give prophylactic indomethacin IV 0.1 mg/kg daily for 3 days — start <12 hours (i.e. 0.08 mg if 800 g etc — be careful writing up the dose)

10 Chest/abdominal X-ray after ETT and umbilical lines; repeat the next day to recheck UVC position — sometimes they migrate (in). Repeat X-ray daily until UVC tip is in a stable position.

11 Clean neck with triclosan swab, then dry; apply a transparent, bio-occlusive, polyurethane dressing (such as Bioclusive, Tegaderm, Opsite); commence topical and enteral nystatin.

12 Monitor serum electrolytes with blood gases. Laboratory specimen for albumin, phosphate twice a week only.

13 Full blood count and film examination (FBC) on days 1, 3, 5 and 7; then twice weekly for 2 weeks; then weekly (with reticulocytes).

14 Cranial ultrasound on days 3, 10 and 42 is recommended as routine. Other units have different regimens; however, it is important to do early scan/s to detect intraventricular haemorrhage and a late scan (≥4 weeks) to detect cystic periventricular leucomalacia.

15 Commence parenteral nutrition on day 3 (via a correctly positioned UVC) if electrolytes stable (especially [K^+] <5 mmol/L).

— Intralipid 20%: 10 mL/kg/day, with Vitalipid N 4 mL/kg/day.

— Commence enteral phosphate if [PO_4^{3-}] is <1.0 mmol/L (see dose page 76).
We rarely need to do this now since we have put more phosphate in our parenteral nutrition.

— Soluvit N: 2 mL/kg Mon–Wed–Fri added to burette with parenteral nutrition line changes.

16 Insert a silastic central venous line (CVL) on day 3–7 as indicated, remove UVC then (by day 5 if possible).

17 Remove UAC on day 7–10.

18 Extubate to nasal CPAP, with prior theophylline, when the ventilator rate is ≤20/min.

19 a Commence nasogastric feeds on day 2–3 as able, 1 mL every 3 hours.

- **b** Increase feeds daily, as able, to 2 mL, 3 mL, 4 mL, then 5 mL every 3 hours.
- **c** Change to 4 mL every 2 hours (if 5 mL every 3 hours is tolerated), and then increase by 1 mL every 12 hours.
- **d** Commence iron supplementation (see page 76) if breast milk feeding at day 14. Not needed if formula-fed.
- **e** Fortify feeds when they are well tolerated.

20 Cease parenteral nutrition when feeds at ~180 mL/kg/day.

21 Try suck feeds from 1600 g or 32 weeks, or sooner if baby is keen to suck.

22 Open cot at 1800 g.

23 Give first immunisation at day 56.

24 Home when all suck feeds, gaining weight, open cot and temperature OK.

CHAPTER 15

Jaundice

David Cartwright, Garry Inglis and Mark Davies

Term newborns

Features to be alert for in term newborns with jaundice are:

- jaundice that is obvious in the first 24 hours of life — measure a total serum bilirubin level (SBR) and look for a specific cause (especially haemolysis)
- a positive Coombs' test (now called direct antibody test, DAT)
- Rhesus, O–A or O–B incompatibility
- numbers for total SBR to carry in your head to alert you to jaundice that is possibly not physiological and may need further investigation at various ages are:
  - 150 µmol/L at 24 hours
  - 200 µmol/L at 48 hours
  - 250 µmol/L at 72 hours
  - 300 µmol/L at any time.

Note: for SBR 1mg/dL ≅ 17 µmol/L.

Investigate babies who need phototherapy:

- Do a 'haemolytic screen' which should include:
  - full blood count and film with reticulocyte count — for red blood cell (RBC) morphology, pyknocytes, spherocytes, etc, and evidence of RBC turnover
  - maternal and baby blood group (if not already known)
  - Heinz bodies
  - DAT (Coombs' test)
  - glucose-6-phosphate dehydrogenase (G6PD) level.
- Order a conjugated SBR separately if you are concerned.
- Order liver function tests separately if concerned. Concerns include severe hyperbilirubinaemia, evidence

of congenital viral infection, green-looking jaundice, pale stools and dark urine.

- Always measure another total SBR a few hours after a high SBR so that you can gauge the rate of rise (or fall if treated).

Therapy guidelines for term newborns

There are no rigorously tested guidelines for therapy. Consider using Figures 15.1 and 15.2 — they are based on experience rather than any rigid testing scheme or randomised controlled trial.

[These graphs were prepared by using data from: Anonymous. Clinical practice guideline: management of hyperbilirubinemia in the newborn infant 35 or more weeks of gestation. American Academy of Pediatrics Subcommittee on Hyperbilirubinemia. Pediatrics 2004;114:297–316 (erratum appears in Pediatrics 2004;114:1138).]

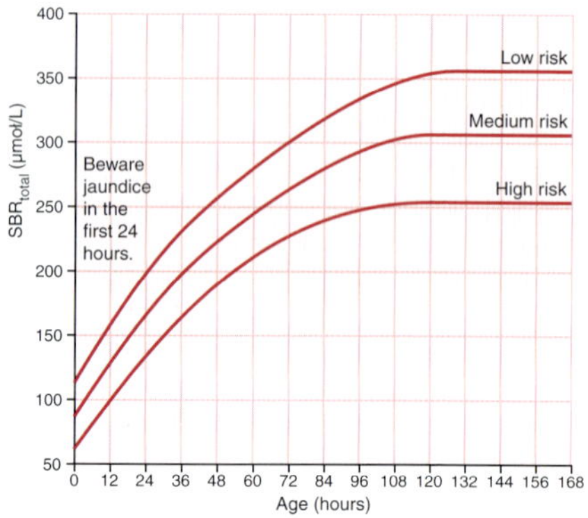

Figure 15.1 Guidelines for phototherapy in infants ≥35 weeks gestational age — if the total SBR plots above the appropriate line, then start intensive phototherapy

SBR_{total} = total serum bilirubin level

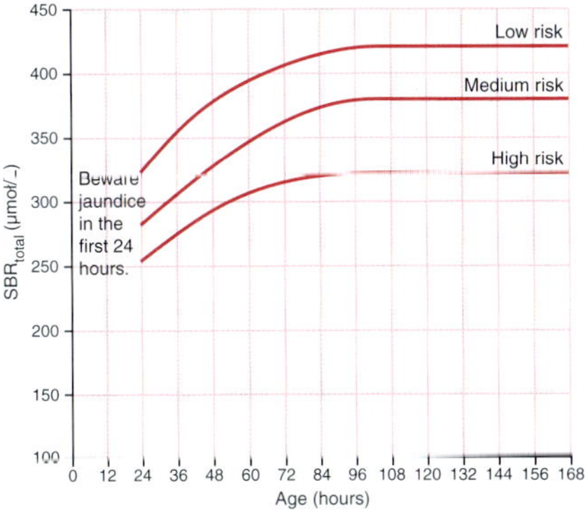

Figure 15.2 Guidelines for exchange transfusion in infants ≥35 weeks gestational age — if the total SBR plots above the appropriate line despite intensive phototherapy, then do an exchange transfusion SBR_{total} = total serum bilirubin level

Low risk: ≥38 weeks gestation and no risk factors.

Medium risk: 35–37^{+6} weeks gestation and no risk factors, OR ≥38 weeks and risk factors present.

High risk: 35–37^{+6} weeks gestation and risk factors present.

`Risk factors: isoimmune haemolytic disease/positive DAT, septicaemia, significant metabolic acidosis, G6PD deficiency, asphyxia, temperature instability, significant lethargy, hypoalbuminaemia.

(DAT = direct antibody test; G6PD = glucose-6-phosphate dehydrogenase)

Preterm newborns

Similar principles apply as for term babies.

Treatment without a haemolytic screen may be started in the right context, especially in those babies who are already having haematological evaluations.

Therapy guidelines for preterm newborns

- For babies <2000 g consider using Figures 15.3 and 15.4.

  [These graphs were prepared by using data from: Cockington RA, Drew JH, Eberhard A. Outcomes following the use of rational guidelines in the management of jaundiced newborn infants. Australian Paediatric Journal 1989;25(6):346–350.]
- It is sometimes useful in very small babies (<1500 g) to consider phototherapy when the serum bilirubin in μmol/L is 10% of the body weight in grams. However, phototherapy is not usually needed with a SBR of <100 μmol/L unless it is rising rapidly.

Prolonged jaundice

- Infants that are jaundiced >10 days in a term infant, >14 days in a preterm infant, also require investigation:

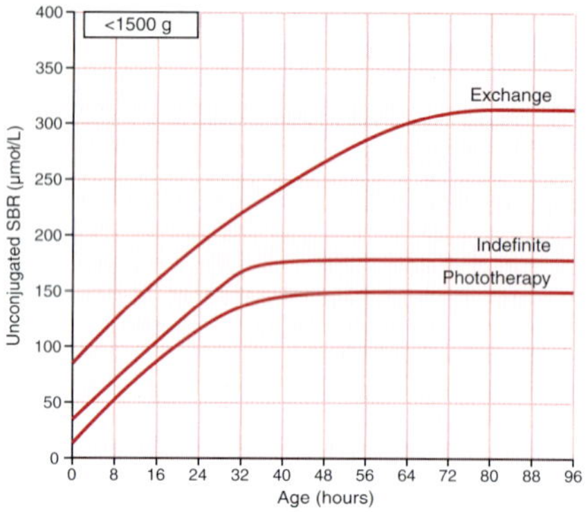

Figure 15.3 Guidelines for treating jaundice in babies <1500 g — if the total SBR plots above the phototherapy line, then start intensive phototherapy; if above either of the other lines, discuss with a consultant neonatologist

SBR = serum bilirubin level

— a 'haemolytic screen' as above
— a total **and** a conjugated SBR
— thyroid function tests (TFTs).

- Always check the maternal and baby blood groups when evaluating jaundice.
  In some hospitals the baby's group and a Coombs' test are routinely performed on cord blood, with the result available the day after birth.
- For conjugated hyperbilirubinaemia, check for alpha-1-antitrypsin deficiency and cystic fibrosis, and order a liver ultrasound: biliary atresia and choledochal cysts are important causes of obstructive jaundice as they are potentially treatable.
- A well baby with normal investigations (as above) will most likely have breast milk jaundice, which is benign.

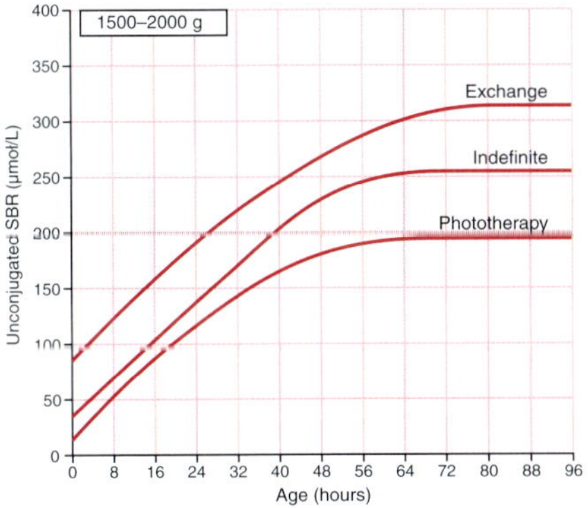

Figure 15.4 Guidelines for treating jaundice in babies 1500–2000 g — if the total SBR plots above the phototherapy line, then start intensive phototherapy; if above either of the other lines discuss with a consultant neonatologist
SBR = serum bilirubin level

Phototherapy

Light in the blue part of the spectrum causes configurational and structural isomerisation of the bilirubin molecule. The structural isomer lumirubin forms the majority of the excreted product, and is excreted via the bile ducts (80%) and the urine (20%). Once formed in the blood it is still measured in standard bilirubin tests, but is no longer lipid-soluble and therefore no longer dangerous to the brain, so phototherapy is helpful even before it has lowered the serum bilirubin level.

To increase the effectiveness of phototherapy:

- Have lights with the right wavelength of light:
  - blue (425–475 nm) or 'special blue': most efficient, but unpleasant to work around
  - green: greater skin penetration
  - white: slightly less efficient than special blue but better to work around.
- Expose greatest possible area of skin:
  - take the nappy off!
  - place lights from the side as well as above, and below with a phototherapy blanket (e.g. biliblanket).
- Increase brightness of lights / closeness to skin — quartz halogen lamps are **very** good because of their high intensity.

> **Remember:**
> Spectral irradiance is measured in
> micro-watts / cm^2 / nm
> This helps you remember
> Intensity / Exposed area / Wavelength

Exchange transfusion

- The decision to do an exchange transfusion is always made by the consultant.
- The method chosen may be:
  - a venous 'push-pull' technique via a size 5FG or 8FG UVC (single operator)

— a continuous technique via a UAC/UVC, UAC/IV, IA/UVC or peripheral IA/IV combination (this requires two operators simultaneously withdrawing and infusing blood).

(IA = intra-arterial line; IV = intravenous line; UAC = umbilical arterial catheter; UVC – umbilical venous catheter.)

- Blood as fresh as possible (<5 days old) should be used.
- You will be supplied with packed cells to be diluted with either fresh frozen plasma (FFP) or 4–5% albumin.
- To calculate the volume of fluid (4–5% albumin or FFP) to add to a bag of packed cells to lower the haematocrit for exchange transfusion, see box below.

Red cell volume supplied = Red cell volume after dilution

Definitions:

- HctB = Haematocrit of bag as supplied — use 0.62, or measure
- HctD = Desired haematocrit, e.g. ~0.50 would be OK
- BagVol = Volume of fluid in bag supplied (weigh it to get a reasonable approximation)
- AddVol = Volume of 4% or 5% albumin or fresh frozen plasma to add to the bag

Calculation:

$$\text{AddVol} = \text{BagVol} \times \left(\frac{\text{HctB}}{\text{HctD}} - 1\right)$$

So, to calculate the added volume required:

- take the supplied haematocrit
  e.g. 0.62
- divide it by the desired haematocrit (the resulting number will always be greater than 1)
  e.g. 0.62 ÷ 0.5 = 1.24
- subtract 1
  e.g. 1.24 – 1 = 0.24
- multiply this by the volume of the bag as supplied
  e.g. 0.24 × 480 = 115.2 mL.

CHAPTER 16

Anaemia and blood product transfusions

Mark Davies and David Cartwright

Anaemia of prematurity

Newborn infants have decreased red blood cell (RBC) production and their haemoglobin concentration [Hb] falls in the weeks/months following birth. This normal fall in Hb is exaggerated in the preterm infant because of decreased erythropoietin production, decreased RBC survival, and blood loss due to frequent blood sampling. This results in anaemia of prematurity: common in preterm infants and universal in extremely low birth weight (ELBW) infants.

The clinical effects of anaemia include:

- increased respiratory effort or shortness of breath
- oxygen requirement not due to other obvious cause (such as chronic lung disease)
- poor weight gain.

When recovery from anaemia of prematurity occurs, iron stores are depleted quickly. **Iron treatment** is used to aid recovery from anaemia of prematurity (see page 76).

Erythropoietin has not been reliably demonstrated to prevent anaemia of prematurity or RBC donor exposure.

Top-up transfusion

- Always get consent for transfusion from parents before administering, and note this in the chart.
- Blood for neonatal 'top-up' transfusions is supplied in paediatric packs (paed packs). A single unit of donor RBC is split into 4 packs averaging ~50 mL (25–100 mL). When a baby uses one of the 4 packs, the

other 3 may be set aside for possible future use in that baby, thus limiting the number of donors the baby may be exposed to.

- The blood supplied in the paed packs has a haematocrit of about 0.6 (0.5–0.7). The blood is filtered to remove 99.998% of white cells, and irradiated.
- Indications:
  - Capillary [Hb] <80 g/L and symptomatic in recovering babies. Some use the haematocrit as a guide — e.g. <0.25–0.3. However, using Hb is better because you are considering the oxygen-carrying capacity of the blood, which correlates more closely to the Hb concentration.
  - Blood may be given at higher [Hb] in more acutely ill babies.
  - Beware of the differences between capillary, venous and arterial Hb measurements. Arterial [Hb] may be 30 g/L below capillary [Hb]; venous [Hb] is in between (Starling's hypothesis of capillary return).
- **Dose: usual volume given is 25–30 mL/kg, over 4–6 hours.**

  Many would transfuse with smaller volumes: this is OK if the haematocrit of the transfused blood is higher (~0.8); however, if not, the actual amount of transfused RBC will be inadequate and more transfusions may be required. This may increase the number of donors that any particular baby is exposed to.

Platelets

Thrombocytopaenia is a common problem in neonates. A cause should be looked for. It may be due to infection, thrombosis, ischaemic gut or isoimmunisation (neonatal alloimmune thrombocytopaenia — can be severe and cause devastating intracranial bleeds).

- Give a platelet transfusion if the platelet count is <25 × 10^9/L. Always get consent for transfusion from parents before administering, and note this in the chart.

- Platelet transfusion may be required at higher platelet counts if there is bleeding or the baby requires surgery or other vascular procedures (e.g. central venous line insertion).
- In alloimmune thrombocytopaenia you may need specially matched platelets (although do not wait for them if there is bleeding). Diagnosis is made by testing both parents' platelet groups for incompatibility. Intravenous immunoglobulin is sometimes used for refractory alloimmune thrombocytopaenia.
- **Dose: usual volume given is 10 mL/kg, over 0.5–1 hour.**

Albumin

The use of albumin infusions for infants with hypoalbuminaemia is controversial.

- Many ELBW infants (especially those whose main nutrition source is parenteral) do not make albumin well. It is these infants who some believe may benefit from an albumin infusion if the serum albumin is <25 g/L.
    - If used, usually 1–2 g/kg of 20% (or 25%) albumin is given over at least 4 hours.
- An infusion of albumin may increase intravascular volume. This may lead to cardiovascular compromise if the albumin is infused too quickly.
  Some clinicians would give frusemide half-way through the infusion to pre-empt this.
- Beware if there are leaky capillaries, as one might see in babies with capillary leak syndrome (CLS) secondary to septicaemia or trauma/surgery. Any infused albumin will leak into the tissues, osmotically dragging fluid with it — making any oedema worse. This may also deplete intravascular volume.

CHAPTER 17

Infection risk

David Cartwright, Mark Davies and Garry Inglis

Infection risk and signs

All babies born after labour or ruptured membranes, either vaginally or by caesarean section, should be regarded as **potentially infected** — regardless of your supposed knowledge of maternal colonisation status.

Risks of infection increase with:

- prolonged rupture of membranes, especially ≥18 hours
- multiple vaginal examinations
- known colonisation with pathogenic organisms, e.g. group B *Streptococcus* (GBS)
- a previously affected infant with early-onset septicaemia.

Signs of infection before delivery may include:

- maternal fever ≥38°C
- maternal tachycardia
- fetal tachycardia
- premature rupture of membranes
- preterm labour.

Signs of infection after birth may include:

- unexpected need for resuscitation
- early onset of apnoea
- fever
- poor peripheral perfusion
- respiratory distress.

Haematological evidence of infection includes:

- neutropaenia
- a left shift — immature : total (IT) neutrophil ratio ≥0.2

- toxic changes seen in neutrophils (toxic granulations, vacuolation, Dohle bodies, intracellular bacteria).

Antibiotic use

There is no magic formula that tells us which babies must be treated with antibiotics.

- If a baby is infected, early treatment is essential. This means treating all babies with reasonable risks, as above, with antibiotics for 36–48 hours until the blood culture is negative (with no haematological evidence of infection) and the baby is known to be well.
- **Treat all babies with respiratory distress with antibiotics** — the only possible exception is those babies born by 'cold' elective Caesarean section or a Caesarean section for pre-eclampsia or intrauterine growth restriction.
- **Treat all babies whose mother has had fever ≥38°C with antibiotics.**
- **Treat all babies born after preterm labour with antibiotics**, unless they are completely well and there are no other risk factors.

> **!** Antibiotics should be given within half an hour of a decision to start them.
>
> Always take a blood culture before commencing antibiotics.
>
> Arrange a full blood count (FBC) and film examination for the next convenient blood collection time.

For early septicaemia

The most common organisms to cover are group B β-haemolytic *Streptococcus* (GBS), *Escherichia coli* and other coliforms.

Antibiotics of first choice are:

- a **penicillin** — e.g. IV penicillin; and
- an **aminoglycoside** or a **3rd-generation cephalosporin** — e.g. IV gentamicin.

For suspected late-onset or nosocomial infection (appearing >48 hours after nursery admission)

Late-onset infection can present in many ways (including signs common in babies without infection), therefore any concerns about an infant should prompt the question: Could this be due to infection? Always err on the side of taking cultures and starting antibiotics.

Common signs include:

- lethargy
- increasing frequency and severity of apnoea and/or desaturation episodes
- change in respiratory status
- gut stasis
- temperature instability
- hypo- or hyperglycaemia
- 'not herself', etc.

The basic principle is to cover:

- possible infecting organisms (including known colonising organisms) — e.g. babies with in situ devices, such as central venous lines, will be more prone to infection with coagulase negative staphylococci (e.g. *Staphylococcus epidermidis*); babies with gut problems will be more prone to infection with gut organisms such as enterococcus and coliforms; and/or
- known organisms that cause late infection in your nursery.

This cover will usually include cover for Gram-positive (with e.g. ampicillin, flucloxacillin or a 1st-generation cephalosporin) and Gram-negative (with e.g. gentamicin or a 3rd-generation cephalosporin) organisms. The antibiotics often have a synergistic effect with each other.

- We usually use ampicillin 50 mg/kg every 12 hours and either cefotaxime 50 mg/kg every 12 hours or gentamicin 2.5 mg/kg daily or every 36 hours (see page 80).

Under some circumstances broader coverage is justified. This may include cover for anaerobes or fungi. Some justify the empirical use of vancomycin on the grounds that most of their infecting organisms are coagulase-negative staphylococci. However, using too much vancomycin will one day lead to the emergence of vancomycin-resistant organisms.

Prevention of neonatal early-onset GBS disease (EOGBSD)

The prevention of early-onset GBS disease requires strategies for both the mother and the baby.

There are two obstetric approaches:

- swab all pregnant women late in the 3rd trimester for GBS, and if positive treat mother with intrapartum antibiotic prophylaxis; or
- use intrapartum antibiotic prophylaxis for mothers who have risk factors.

The neonatal approach is outlined below.

Queensland approach

Following consideration of all available information and in the light of the current low rate (0.39/1000 births) of EOGBSD in Queensland in 2002, the Perinatal Clinical Practice Guidelines Working Party on Early Onset Group B Streptococcal Disease and Prelabour Rupture of the Membranes at Term (coordinated by the Centre for Clinical Studies, Mater Hospital, South Brisbane and the Southern Zone Maternal Neonatal and Gynaecology Network, Southern Zone Management Unit) reached a consensus to continue to recommend the modified risk factor approach.

They have produced the *Clinical Practice Guidelines for the prevention of neonatal early-onset group B streptococcal disease (EOGBSD) for Queensland hospitals*.

Our suggested approach in light of these guidelines is:

1. Routine antenatal screening for GBS is not recommended.
2. Intrapartum antibiotic prophylaxis for EOGBSD during the first stage of labour (delivery anticipated within 6 hours) should be offered to:
   - women who have had a previous infant with EOGBSD
   - women who are known to have had a positive GBS culture during this pregnancy from the urinary, genital or lower intestinal tract
   - women who might have >18 hours of ruptured membranes before delivery
   - women in preterm labour at a gestational age of 34 weeks or less (i.e. <35 weeks).
3. Women with an intrapartum fever of ≥38°C or with other indications of chorioamnionitis require broad-spectrum antibiotic treatment (not prophylaxis) and treatment needs to be continued following delivery. The paediatric staff must be notified immediately if a mother shows signs of sepsis within 24 hours of delivery.
4. The antibiotic regimen recommended for intrapartum GBS prophylaxis is:

   penicillin 1.2 g IV load, then 0.6 g IV every 4–6 hours during the course of labour

   or

   - for those women with a history of penicillin allergy, clindamycin 900 mg IV every 8 hours, or erythromycin 500 mg IV every 6 hours until delivery.
5. Units should be familiar with their anaphylaxis protocol.
6. For **all newborns**, follow the Neonatal Sepsis Protocol (Fig 17.1 on page 112; modified from the above guidelines).

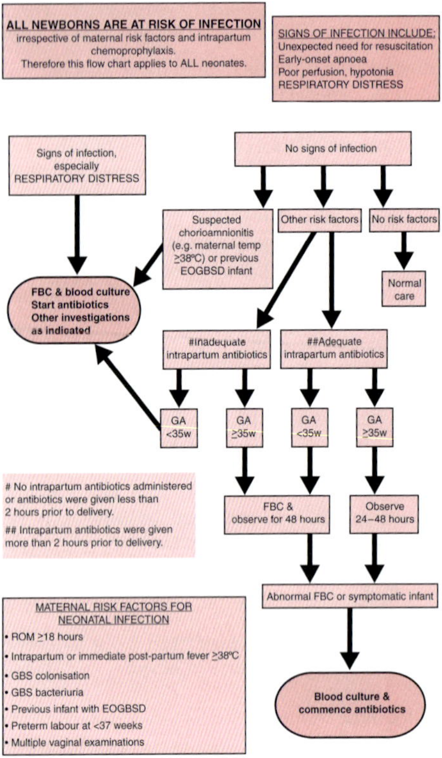

Figure 17.1 Neonatal sepsis protocol
EOGBSD = early-onset GBS disease; FBC = full blood count; GA = gestational age (weeks); GBS = group B *Streptococcus*; ROM = rupture of membranes

CHAPTER 18

Retinopathy of prematurity (ROP)

Mark Davies and Garry Inglis

- The strongest risk factors for ROP are gestation and birth weight. The majority of significant ROP occurs in babies born at less than 28 weeks gestation.
- The association between ROP and oxygen therapy is well documented.
- Many with significant ROP also have chronic lung disease.

Babies at high risk for ROP are examined by an ophthalmologist to screen for the disorder.

- The most commonly used criteria for ROP screening are birth weight <1500 g or gestation at birth <32 weeks (as is done in our unit).
- Some units will include slightly bigger or mature babies if they have required significant oxygen supplementation or have otherwise been significantly unwell.
- Screening should begin at around 31 weeks post-menstrual age or 4 weeks of age.
- Frequency of re-examination will depend upon the findings.

Management

ROP is described according to the retinal zone involved (Zones 1–3), the stage of disease (Stages 1–5), the extent of disease (in clock hours) and whether there is 'plus' disease present.

- In most babies the retina will vascularise progressively from posterior (Zone 1) to anterior (Zone 3) without the need for intervention.
- In a small number, usually those with Stage 3 or greater disease (although the decision will depend on factors such as how aggressive the disease is and will obviously rest with the ophthalmologist), the retinopathy will be treated in an attempt to arrest disease progression and preserve as much functional vision as possible.
- Treatment for 'threshold' retinopathy will usually consist of photocoagulation (laser).
  Less commonly, cryotherapy is used.
- For more advanced disease, treatment may include a scleral buckle procedure or vitrectomy — in reality these are rarely required.

Laser therapy for ROP

Laser may be done under local anaesthetic, general anaesthetic, sedation, or a combination of these. The specific procedure will vary by unit and ophthalmologist but is usually done in the intensive care nursery. A description of the procedure as performed in our unit is provided below.

Suggested laser therapy procedure

The laser treatment is usually done in the intensive care nursery. The infants with severe ROP requiring laser treatment are often babies who were very small and/or very preterm who have had a stormy neonatal course. Most will have, or have had, significant chronic lung disease (CLD).

The ophthalmologist usually requires:

- the laser
- goggles for the laser operator and all staff working in the same room
- a 30D lens
- a small eye-speculum pack

continued

- various eye drops and treatments:
  - amethocaine eye drops
  - cyclopentolate 0.2% / phenylephrine 1% eye drops for pupil dilation
  - balanced salt solution (BSS) — this is not the same as Normal saline, Nsaline (0.9%)
  - dexamethasone 1 mg/mL (Maxidex 0.1%)
  - dorzolamide HCl 2% 20 mg/mL (Trusopt)
  - chloramphenicol ointment (Chlorsig).

Once it is confirmed that the ophthalmologist is actually coming to do the procedure:

- obtain venous access prior to intubation
- give the usual sedation (see pages 29 and 81) plus vecuronium (0.1 mg/kg) for intubation
- Intubate and ventilate just ahead of time
- dilate pupils 30 minutes prior to laser starting
- position baby supine with the head towards the foot of the bed (i.e. the baby's head pointing towards the middle of the room)
- when the ophthalmologist arrives, ensure the baby is sedated and paralysed — e.g. morphine (0.1–0.15 mg/kg) and midazolam (0.1–0.15 mg/kg) and vecuronium (0.1 mg/kg) or pancuronium (0.1 mg/kg).

A neonatologist or other member of the neonatal medical staff stays close by during the entire procedure.

Repeat doses of muscle relaxant may be required.

Monitor the baby's heart rate for evidence of inadequate analgesia.

The baby is usually ventilated overnight and extubated the next morning, if the ventilation has not exacerbated the CLD too much.

CHAPTER 19

Cranial ultrasounds

Mark Davies and David Cartwright

Findings

A routine head ultrasound (US) is recommended for all babies <1750 g or <32 weeks gestational age (GA), on days 3 and 10. A routine late head US is recommended at 6 weeks (or 4 weeks of age if >1200 g).

Different schemes will operate in different hospitals. Some units will do a routine US on day 1. Some will limit routine scans to lower birth weights and GAs.

Intraventricular haemorrhage (IVH)

IVH is graded by the worst IVH on either side.

Grade	Features
1	Germinal matrix or sub-ependymal bleed, no intraventricular blood
2	Grade 1 plus intraventricular blood, no ventricular dilatation
3	Grade 2 plus ventricular dilatation
4	Grade 3 plus haemorrhage in the periventricular area

A Grade 4 bleed is not an extension of a Grade 3 bleed. It is probably a haemorrhagic–ischaemic lesion secondary to venous congestion (venous infarction) in the periventricular region due to the germinal matrix bleed.

Periventricular echogenicity (PVE)

- This may be due to a Grade 4 IVH and may lead to porencephaly.
- When not associated with IVH, it is usually an area of ischaemia/infarction and represents white-matter injury. The US appearance may resolve completely or become cystic periventricular leucomalacia.
- PVE that persists >7–14 days but does not become cystic increases the risk of cerebral palsy (CP) to ~5–10%.

Periventricular leucomalacia (PVL)

- Overall, at least 50% of infants with PVL have cerebral palsy (CP).
- The best outcome is with unilateral frontal cysts — the majority are normal at follow-up.
- The worst outcome is with multiple bilateral parieto-occipital cysts — >90% of survivors have a severe disability.

Outcomes

Table 19.1 on page 118 summarises the outcomes for various cranial US findings.

- Most studies report results from routine ultrasounds done on infants either < ~1500 g birthweight or < ~32–34 weeks GA.
- The studies usually report CP/disability rates in survivors. However, they all report different outcomes that will mean different things.
- Numbers in the 'Outcome' column are either from individual studies or a conglomeration of studies.

Table 19.1 Outcomes for various cranial ultrasound (US) findings in populations of high-risk infants (as detailed in text)

US finding	Outcome
Normal	5–8% have significant motor deficit, IQ <70, and/or moderate/severe disability
Intraventricular haemorrhage, IVH	
1	4–5% severe disability
2	10–15% severe disability
3	20–35% CP/intellectual deficit
4, all	~50–70% CP/intellectual deficit/IQ <70; 30–60% will need VP shunt
4 + cysts	80% moderate/severe disability; 90+% CP
Periventricular echogenicity, PVE (no cysts)	
<7 days	as for normal scan
7–21 days	6–8% CP ±intellectual deficit
>21 days	>80% some neurological abnormality/CP
Periventricular leucomalacia, PVL	
All	50–60% moderate/severe disability; 50–100% CP
Unilateral	40–50% CP
Bilateral	85–95% CP
Focal	50–60% CP
Extensive	>95% CP
Small	60–70% CP
Large	>90% CP
Ventriculomegaly	
PHVD	25–35% moderate/severe disability
	50–60% need VP shunt
Ventriculomegaly at term	45–55% IQ <70; 40–50% CP
Hydrocephalus	50–60% moderate/severe disability
	50–60% need VP shunt
Shunted	40–60% moderate/severe disability

CP = cerebral palsy; IQ = intelligence quotient; PHVD = post-haemorrhagic ventricular dilatation; VP = ventriculo-peritoneal.

CHAPTER 20

Apnoea

David Cartwright and Mark Davies

Background

Definition:

- either 20 seconds of zero flow in or out of the lungs; or
- 10 seconds of zero flow accompanied by desaturation or bradycardia.

An episode of apnoea may or may not be accompanied by bradycardia and cyanosis.

Causes of apnoea in newborns:

- infection — meningitis, septicaemia, pneumonia, necrotising enterocolitis, viral upper respiratory tract infection (especially respiratory syncytial virus, RSV)
- hypoxia
- acidosis
- seizures
- metabolic disturbances — hypoglycaemia, hyponatraemia, hypocalcaemia
- intraventricular haemorrhage
- airway obstruction
- gastric or abdominal distension
- gastro-oesophageal reflux, including lowered pH in mid-oesophagus
- apnoea of prematurity (many of the above may contribute to this).

Consequences of apnoea:

- hypoxia / acidosis
- progressive atelectasis
- gastro-oesophageal reflux
- aspiration.

Investigations may include:

- blood sugar level (BSL), arterial blood gas (ABG), urea and electrolytes (U&Es), calcium, magnesium, blood culture, full blood count (FBC) and film examination
- chest X-ray
- lumbar puncture
- cranial ultrasound examination.

Apnoea of prematurity

- Apnoea occurs because of brain-stem immaturity in babies less than about 34 weeks gestational age.
  - The apnoea is worse the more immature the baby.
  - Apnoea usually starts after 2 days of age.
- Bradycardia and hypotonia may accompany apnoea, or occur independently in the same infant.
- Apnoeic episodes are more common during rapid eye movement (REM) sleep.
  - At 32 weeks gestational age, babies sleep about 18 hr/day, of which 80% is REM sleep.
  - At 3 months of age, they sleep about 14 hr/day, of which 40% is REM sleep.
- Apnoea is more common the higher the environmental temperature, and during feeding or defaecating.
- **Any baby with increasing severity or frequency of apnoea must be considered infected, and covered with antibiotics, until proven otherwise (see Ch 17).**

Management of apnoea

Preventive:

- Prevent hypoxia/acidosis, fluctuations in oxygen requirement, reflux or aspiration.
- Feed slowly, give small volumes, avoid gastric or abdominal distension; prone positioning may help.

Treatment:

- Stimulate early.
- Monitor.

- Drugs:
  - — theophylline/aminophylline (see page 80)
  - — caffeine (see page 80)
  - — doxapram may be added to methylxanthines, but must be given by continuous infusion.
- Mechanical treatment — continuous positive airway pressure (CPAP), ventilation.

Response to theophylline:

- 15% respond at serum level of 4.2 mg/L
- 30% respond at serum level of 8.5 mg/L
- 75% respond at serum level of 12.7 mg/L
- 80% respond at serum level of 15.3 mg/L.

However, there is no need to routinely measure the theophylline level. Both effectiveness and toxicity are very obvious clinically:

1. If a baby's apnoea is controlled on a standard dose and they are not tachycardic, then the baby is either receiving adequate drug or doesn't need any.
2. If a baby is persistently tachycardic on theophylline, then they are toxic by definition, whatever the serum theophylline level might be.
3. If a baby's apnoea is not controlled on a standard dose of theophylline, a serum level may help you to determine whether the drug is not being adequately absorbed, or if the baby is a 'non-responder'.

Theophylline is usually ceased after 34 weeks gestational age if there is no apnoea. Monitoring for apnoea should continue for a few days after ceasing theophylline.

CHAPTER 21

Seizures

Mark Davies and David Cartwright

- Seizures can present as subtle alterations in behaviour or movement (including eyes and/or face); hypoventilation, respiratory pauses or apnoea; or more obvious tonic, clonic or tonic-clonic episodes.
- Seizures are most commonly associated with hypoxic-ischaemic encephalopathy (HIE). In babies with HIE it is also important to control other potential causes of seizures such as hypoglycaemia and hyponatraemia — check blood sugar level (BSL) and urea & electrolytes (U&Es).
- Brief myoclonic jerks are common in preterm infants and do not usually represent seizure activity.

Management

- Seizures usually respond to initial therapy with phenobarbitone given as a bolus dose.
  - Give 20 mg/kg initially.
  - If the seizures are not controlled, then a further 2 to 3 bolus doses of 10 mg/kg may be given.
  - Phenobarbitone may cause respiratory depression at high doses.
- **In HIE**, once seizures are under control, a maintenance dose of phenobarbitone may or may not be started.
- If seizures are not controlled with phenobarbitone, other drugs used include:
  - midazolam
  - clonazepam
  - phenytoin.

  Some clinicians use midazolam as first-line treatment.

Seizures not due to HIE

Apart from HIE, other possible causes include cerebrovascular obstruction or bleeds; infection (e.g. meningitis); hypoglycaemia; derangements of electrolytes (e.g. sodium); unconjugated hyperbilirubinaemia; cerebral malformations; neonatal abstinence syndrome; and rare metabolic conditions.

Check:

- Blood — blood sugar level (BSL), arterial blood gas (ABG), urea & electrolytes (U&Es), calcium, magnesium, blood culture, full blood count (FBC) and film examination.
- Cerebrospinal fluid (CSF) — microscopy and culture (bacterial and viral).
- Cranial ultrasound and possibly computerised tomography (CT) or magnetic resonance imaging (MRI).
- Electroencephalogram (EEG).

Consider other metabolic or infective causes.

CHAPTER 22

Neonatal abstinence syndrome (NAS)

Mark Davies and David Cartwright

[From: Guidelines for the management of babies of substance-using women. Norton B, Kuhnert L et al. Brisbane: Grantley Stable Neonatal Unit; 2001.]

Admission guidelines

Indications for admission to the special care nursery (SCN)

Babies of mothers who have a history of using:

- opiates (heroin, methadone)
- amphetamines (speed, Ritalin) — the evidence for NAS in infants of mothers using amphetamines alone is weak
- benzodiazepines (Serepax, diazepam)
- cocaine (crack).

Admission to the special care nursery (SCN)

1. Babies at risk for NAS are monitored using the Finnegan Neonatal Abstinence Score. The minimum stay is 72 hours.

   Some units allow this monitoring on the postnatal ward.
2. Baby is then transferred to postnatal ward (until at least 5 days of age) to be with mother.

Pharmacological treatment

Commence pharmacological treatment once the Finnegan scores average >8 for three consecutive scores or average >12 for two consecutive scores. Pharmacological treatment should always be done in the special care nursery.

Morphine

Morphine is used for opiate withdrawal, e.g. methadone, heroin, pethidine.

- **Dose:**
  - — start at 0.5 mg/kg/day orally, given every 6 hours (0.125 mg/kg/dose).
  - — increase by 0.1 mg/kg/day orally daily until controlled or until dose is 1 mg/kg/day.
- If the baby is requiring 0.9 mg/kg/day or more to control withdrawal symptoms, it is necessary to monitor cardio-respiratory function.
  Consider addition of phenobarbitone 5 mg/kg/day if still not controlled on 1 mg/kg/day of morphine.
- **Weaning** — reduce dose by 0.1 mg/kg/day every 4 days or longer.
- If baby vomits the dose within 5 minutes, it may be readministered once only.

Phenobarbitone

Phenobarbitone is used for non-opioid withdrawal

- **Dose:**
  - — Start with a loading dose of 15 mg/kg — IV/oral (oral dose to be given via a nasogastric tube due to large volume).
    Then start a maintenance dose of 5–10 mg/kg/day (in two divided doses), starting 12 hours after the loading dose. If 10 mg/kg/day is used it should be decreased to 5 mg/kg/day after 48 hours.
  - — If <10 mg/kg/day is used, then the dose can be increased by 2 mg/kg/day until NAS is controlled or the dose is at 10 mg/kg/day. Then decrease after 48 hours at this dose.

- **Weaning** — reduce the dose by 2–4 mg/kg/day every 3 days (or longer depending on the baby's response).
- If the baby vomits the dose within 5 minutes, then it may be repeated once only.

Breastfeeding

- Heroin use — breastfeeding is contraindicated.
- Methadone — breastfeeding is encouraged.
- Methadone plus other drugs — breastfeeding is not recommended.
- Hepatitis C — temporarily discontinue breastfeeding if nipples become cracked or bleed. Express and discard milk until completely healed.
- Women who are HIV-positive should not breastfeed.

On discharge

Infants at risk for NAS may be at risk of significant social problems when discharged — these issues should be explored prior to discharge with the involvement of a social worker.

CHAPTER 23

Surgical problems

Mark Davies and Garry Inglis

Bile

Bile may appear in vomitus or in aspirates from gastric tubes. Bilious vomiting should always be considered as potentially serious, especially in a previously well baby when an acute volvulus should be suspected and ruled out.

Generally speaking, the presence of bile that has made its way into the stomach (and is seen in vomitus or gastric tube aspirates) indicates that the gut is obstructed. This obstruction may be complete or partial, and may be anatomical or functional (i.e. with a still patent lumen).

For **anatomical causes of obstruction** see pages 131–3.

Functional gut obstruction can occur in babies in the following circumstances:

- gastrointestinal perforation (see below)
- necrotising enterocolitis (NEC; see below)
- post-surgical
- any baby that is generally unwell (especially with infection)
- gut immaturity, especially in babies <30–32 weeks gestational age.

Sometimes bile is seen in aspirates when the feeding tube sits at or has passed through the pylorus — this can be confirmed on an abdominal X-ray. In an otherwise well baby, this can be fixed by pulling the tube back so that its tip lies in the body of the stomach.

Determining cause

Significant causes of bile vomiting or bile-stained aspirates need to be distinguished from benign causes (such as a malplaced nasogastric tube or gut immotility due to immaturity) by examining the baby, and doing an abdominal X-ray and a full blood count (FBC) and film examination (and taking a blood culture and starting antibiotics if there is any suspicion of infection).

- **Benign causes** will usually be found in babies who are otherwise well with a soft, non-distended, non-tender abdomen that is not discoloured, who are passing normal stools.
- **Significant causes** may be associated with one or more of:
  - — an unwell baby
  - — an abnormal abdominal exam — distended, tender or tense, discolouration, mass, absent bowel sounds
  - — an abnormal abdominal X-ray — evidence of gastrointestinal perforation or necrotising enterocolitis, fluid levels, bowel distension
  - — an abnormal FBC — signs of infection, thrombocytopaenia.

Gastrointestinal perforation

Extremely preterm infants are prone to gastrointestinal perforation, which can occur in isolation or, more commonly, in association with necrotising enterocolitis (NEC; see below). If intestinal perforation is found, it does not automatically follow that NEC is present. It can be difficult to distinguish the two conditions pre-operatively, and risk factors are similar.

- Clinically the abdomen with perforated bowel and hence free peritoneal gas is almost always 'smooth' in appearance. When bowel loops are visible through the abdominal wall, often described as a 'ropey' abdomen, free gas is usually not present.
- In a plain supine X-ray of the abdomen, the presence of free gas in the peritoneal cavity (pneumoperitoneum) is

demonstrated as a grey outline around the abdominal edge, with the falciform ligament visible in the upper abdomen to the right of the midline. This gas shadow is sometimes called the 'football' sign. Remember that the plain abdominal film is not usually taken erect, so don't waste your time looking for a rim of free gas under the diaphragm. If in doubt, a right-side-up lateral decubitus film may be helpful as the gas may rise above the right lobe of the liver.

- 'Double-shadowing' of bowel walls is also indicative of free gas in the abdominal cavity — the Frimann-Dahl sign or Rigler's sign. Normally only the mucosal surface of the bowel is contrasted by the presence of gas; free gas abutting the serosal surface creates another interface, giving rise to the characteristic double-shadow.
- Suspicion of free gas within the peritoneal cavity should also be raised where an unusually shaped shadow is present — i.e. if the gas shadow does not conform to any anatomical structure.

The **management of infants with gastrointestinal perforation** should include:

- stopping enteral feeds
- nasogastric tube with regular aspiration
- intravenous fluids
- antibiotics (after blood culture)
- immediate review by a paediatric surgeon; encourage them to do a laparotomy.

Necrotising enterocolitis (NEC)

This inflammatory disorder of the bowel has multifactorial causes. The extremely preterm infant is at greater risk.

There is a wide spectrum of clinical features in NEC. **Signs** can include feeding intolerance, vomiting, lethargy, temperature instability, abdominal distension, diarrhoea with or without frank blood, abdominal wall erythema and shock.

The Bell criteria are often used to classify the severity of the illness:

- **Stage 1** — suspected NEC (generally unwell with feed intolerance and/or non-specific abdominal signs, ±bloody stool, but no pneumatosis)
- **Stage 2** — definite NEC (unwell with definite abdominal signs and pneumatosis)
- **Stage 3** — advanced NEC (severely ill with shock, marked abdominal signs, and ascites or intestinal perforation).

In general terms, large-bowel NEC is a much more benign illness than small-bowel NEC.

The characteristic **radiographic findings** are pneumatosis intestinalis and portal venous gas. Pneumatosis intestinalis represents gas in the submucous layer produced by intestinal bacteria.

- There are three patterns of pneumatosis intestinalis:
  - the circle of submucous gas in a cross-section of bowel viewed end on;
  - a 'tram-track' appearance of submucous gas in bowel viewed in longitudinal section; and
  - a 'whorl' pattern seen when looking through a bowel wall with pneumatosis in it.
- Submucosal gas is sometimes absorbed into the portal venous system and travels to the liver, where it can be evident on a plain radiograph. It can also be detected with real-time ultrasound.
- Other radiographic signs to look for in NEC are generalised or local distension from ileus, separation of bowel loops by extra intraperitoneal fluid, and pneumoperitoneum from perforation (see section on intestinal perforation).

Treatment of NEC consists of:

- stopping enteral feeds
- nasogastric tube with regular aspiration
- intravenous fluids
- antibiotics (after blood culture) — traditionally ampicillin, gentamicin and metronidazole

- frequent clinical review
- surgical intervention — evidence of perforation or ischaemic bowel (e.g. a persistent dilated loop) is an absolute indication for this.

Gut obstruction — anatomical causes

Gut obstructions are usually anatomical and congenital. The presenting features of gut obstruction will depend on the anatomical level of the obstruction. In general: the higher the obstruction, the earlier is the presentation; and the lower the obstruction, the more impressive is the abdominal distension.

Some obstructions (e.g. oesophageal atresia, imperforate anus, duodenal atresia) are often associated with other congenital anomalies or may occur as part of recognised syndromes (e.g. VATER, CHARGE, Down syndrome). Many anatomical obstructions, particularly those in the mid to lower small bowel, are thought to result from in-utero vascular events. Also, the presence of one gut atresia makes a second atresia more likely in the same baby. Always examine the baby carefully for associated anomalies.

Oesophageal atresia

Oesophageal obstructions often present with difficulty feeding and the baby is frequently described as being excessively 'mucusy'.

- If oesophageal atresia is suspected, insert a large (8–10FG) tube into the oesophageal pouch. The tube will stop at around 10 cm from the mouth. A narrow tube may coil in the upper oesophageal pouch without resistance being felt, which can falsely lead to the assumption that the oesophagus is patent. Always obtain a chest and abdominal X-ray.
- Some like to perform an air oesophagogram to demonstrate the oesophageal pouch: inject 20 mL of air quickly as the X-ray exposure is made.

- The presence of gas in the stomach indicates that a distal tracheo-oesophageal fistula is present.
- Mechanical ventilation may result in distension of the stomach via the fistula, which can result in gastric rupture.
  - Ventilate as gently as possible and request an early paediatric surgical review.
  - Insert a large-bore catheter (e.g. a Replogle tube) for continuous suction, nurse prone and give parenteral fluids.
  - Almost all infants will have residual problems with gastro-oesophageal reflux and oesophageal dysmotility.

Proximal bowel obstruction

Proximal intestinal obstructions present with early onset of vomiting and distension of the upper abdomen. The vomiting may be bile-stained or non-bile-stained, depending on whether the obstruction is distal or proximal to the ampulla of Vater.

Pyloric stenosis

Pyloric stenosis is uncommon in neonates. It causes non-bile-stained 'projectile' vomiting.

- If suspected, examine for a palpable pyloric tumour and visible upper abdominal peristaltic waves.
- Ultrasound examination can be used to measure the length and thickness of the pyloric muscle.
- Intravenous fluids may be needed.
- Check arterial blood gas (ABG) and electrolytes.

Duodenal atresia

Duodenal atresia presents soon after birth with persistent vomiting, which is usually bile-stained.

- Insert a nasogastric tube and aspirate — there will usually be a large volume of fluid.
- Give intravenous fluids. Monitor electrolytes.
- On a plain supine radiograph there will be a J-shaped shadow, representative of gas in a distended stomach and

duodenum, with absence of gas more distally. The typical 'double bubble' is demonstrated on an erect film.

- Paediatric surgical intervention is required.

Jejunal/ileal atresia

Distal small-bowel atresia presents later than duodenal atresia. Bile-stained vomiting and abdominal distension are typical. With more distal obstructions, fluid and electrolyte disturbance at presentation is more likely.

Malrotation

Malrotation with volvulus can present from soon after birth to several months later. Features include bile-stained vomiting and variable abdominal distension. If the mesenteric vascular supply is compromised the infant can rapidly progress to peritonitis and shock, with gangrene of the bowel.

- This is a **medical emergency** that must be recognised and treated urgently to avoid potentially catastrophic ischaemic bowel injury.
- A plain abdominal radiograph may show a dilated stomach and proximal duodenum. The appearance of a malrotation with volvulus can be indistinguishable from that of duodenal atresia. However, the latter can be excluded by the appearance of gas more distal to the obstruction.
- An upper gastrointestinal contrast study can be useful in defining the nature of the obstruction, but do not allow this to delay a paediatric surgeon seeing the baby.
- Start intravenous fluids and antibiotics. Many will require parenteral nutrition.

Baby of mother with polyhydramnios

The cause of polyhydramnios is usually not known. It can be associated with maternal conditions such as diabetes or pre-eclampsia.

- In most instances where there is an underlying fetal cause it should be fairly obvious clinically once the baby is born. As you examine the baby, think of why he/she might have had reduced fetal swallowing or increased urine output.

- The most commonly identified cause is upper gastrointestinal obstruction (especially oesophageal or duodenal atresia — see above). Can you pass a feeding tube into the stomach?
- Central nervous system defects (e.g. anencephaly, neuromuscular disorders affecting swallowing) should be quite obvious, as should abdominal wall defects, severe skeletal dysplasias and chromosomal abnormalities.
- Examine the infant for evidence of respiratory tract abnormalities (e.g. congenital cyst-adenomatoid malformation), congenital diaphragmatic hernia or cardiac anomalies.
- Polyhydramnios may be associated with hydrops fetalis. In multiple gestation, consider twin–twin transfusion syndrome.
- Monitor urine output to check for polyuric renal disorders.

Delayed passage of meconium

The normal time to passage of meconium increases with decreasing gestational age (GA).

- At term, first passage of meconium should occur by 48 hours.
- Below 32 weeks GA, up to half may not pass meconium until beyond 48 hours, and some may take up to 10 days.

Common causes of delayed passage of meconium include anorectal malformations, Hirschsprung disease and meconium ileus. All can present also with vomiting and abdominal distension.

Diagnosis

Always examine the perineum and anus carefully.

- The finding of meconium in the nappy does not exclude anal atresia, as it is often associated with a recto-perineal, recto-vesical or recto-vaginal fistula. An 'anal' dimple, usually more anterior than normal, can be mistaken for an anus but the diagnosis of this condition need not be difficult.

— If imperforate anus is present, abdominal X-ray will often show dilated bowel with or without gas in the rectum, depending on the length of the atretic segment.
— Keep 'nil by mouth' and give intravenous fluids.
— Check for associated anomalies.
— Seek specialist neonatal and paediatric surgical advice.

- The diagnosis of Hirschsprung disease may be more difficult. These infants usually have delayed passage of meconium with or without vomiting and abdominal distension. In milder cases there may be a history of recurrent constipation.
  — If suspected, get an abdominal X-ray, which may show dilated loops of bowel but is generally non-specific. Likewise, a lower bowel contrast study is also generally not specific for any particular diagnosis. However, if contrast material is still present on a late film (24 hours after the contrast study), it makes Hirschsprung disease the most likely diagnosis, as normal bowel motility would usually evacuate the contrast material quickly after such a study.
  — The typical appearance of a narrowed distal segment with more proximal dilatation may not become apparent in the neonatal period. Rectal suction biopsy is usually performed to confirm absence of ganglion cells prior to more definitive repair — seek paediatric surgical advice.
  — If the baby is unwell, stop feeds, check electrolytes, give intravenous fluids and give antibiotics.
- Meconium ileus is suggested by the delayed passage of (thick, inspissated) meconium, with or without abdominal distension and vomiting.

— The abdominal X-ray often shows dilated loops of bowel but with an absence or paucity of gas in the right iliac fossa due to the presence of the inspissated meconium, which can appear granular.
— A contrast enema may show a microcolon, indicating that the colon has not had any solid contents in it for a long time, and may be effective in relieving the obstruction.
— Complicated meconium ileus (e.g. volvulus, atresia, perforation) will require surgical intervention.

Gastroschisis

The major risks to the infant with gastroschisis are compromised circulation to the gut, gut obstruction, loss of heat and water from the exposed bowel, and infection.

Therefore, the important aspects of the immediate management of a baby born with gastroschisis are:

- Manage any respiratory problems as for babies without gastroschisis — some surgeons would prefer that you avoid nasal continuous positive airway pressure (CPAP).
- Make sure that the external bowel is not twisted on itself (usually occurs at the abdominal wall defect).
- Support the gut so that the external bowel is not being stretched.
- Cover the bowel — either put baby in a 'bowel bag' up to the chest, or cover with polyethylene kitchen-wrap/cling-wrap.
- Insert a nasogastric tube, leave on free drainage and aspirate every 15 minutes.
- Intravenous antibiotics (metronidazole, gentamicin, penicillin).
- Maintenance intravenous fluids.

Call a paediatric surgeon prior to delivery if the diagnosis was made antenatally, otherwise call them as soon as you can after the baby is stabilised.
The sooner the gut is reduced, the better.

Congenital diaphragmatic hernia (CDH)

The diagnosis is usually known before birth. If not, it should be suspected immediately after birth in a baby who requires resuscitation with initial respiratory distress, rapid deterioration (cyanosis, bradycardia, pallor), poor response to resuscitation, right-sided heart sounds (if a left CDH) and a scaphoid abdomen.

Immediate management should include:

- Intubation and ventilation.
- Insert a gastric tube to empty stomach of air (and keep empty).
- Surfactant.
- Sedation (morphine and midazolam).
- Admit to the intensive care nursery.
- Ongoing ventilation is managed as for pulmonary hypertension (see p 60).
- Surgery to close the diaphragm and relocate the abdominal contents should be delayed for a few days until the baby is stable.

The primary problem in CDH is the pulmonary hypoplasia. In babies with a left-sided hernia (~85%), there is gross hypoplasia of the left lung and significant hypoplasia of the right lung — surgery will not cure this. The hypoplastic lungs have a reduced number of poorly formed peripheral air spaces and abnormal pulmonary vasculature. This results in poor ventilation and severely restricted pulmonary blood flow.

CHAPTER 24

Maternal thyroid disease

Mark Davies

Abnormalities of thyroid function in the newborn infant can result from maternal thyroid disease. This can be due to maternal antithyroid antibodies transferred from the mother (thyroid-stimulating antibodies or thyroid-blocking antibodies, or both), the state of maternal thyroid function during the pregnancy, or any treatment the mother has had for her thyroid disease during the pregnancy.

The maternal thyroid disease does not need to be active to cause problems for the baby; the mother may still have circulating antibodies.

- Therefore all babies whose mothers have thyroid disease, or a past history of thyroid disease, should have thyroid function tests (TFTs) — including thyroid-stimulating hormone (TSH/thyrotropin) and free thyroxine (FT4) — done at 4–5 days old. Beware checking earlier as the TSH is higher in the first day or two of life.
- Infants of mothers with uncontrolled hyperthyroidism should also have repeat TFTs at 2 weeks of age.
- Any infant with signs or symptoms of hypo- or hyperthyroidism should have TFTs done.

CHAPTER 25

Hips

David Cartwright

Examination for congenital hip dysplasia and dislocation of the hip (now known as developmental dysplasia of the hip, DDH) is an important part of the assessment of normal newborns. This condition is more common in females.

Particular attention should also be paid to:

- breech presentations, especially those with extended legs
- babies with features of in-utero compression such as calcaneovalgus foot deformities, talipes equinovarus, asymmetry of lower jaw, marked head moulding
- babies from pregnancies with oligohydramnios.

Most information will be gained by performing the examination as soon as possible after birth. It **must** also be done again before discharge, and should be done whenever a baby in the first few months of life is seen, for whatever reason.

You are examining to determine four kinds of hips:

- normal
- dislocatable hip, reduced at rest
- dislocated hip, reducible by manipulation
- dislocated hip, not reducible (fixed dislocation).

Examination of the hips

1. Stand at the foot end of the cot.
2. Observe the position and spontaneous movements of the hips with the nappy removed.
   A dislocated hip is held in a slightly adducted and flexed position.

3 Gently take the lower legs in your hands, with your thumbs pointing towards the knees.
Compare the lengths of the femurs by approximating the knees to the midline, without applying any backwards or forwards pressure, with the hips and the knees each flexed to 90°. The femur with a dislocated hip will appear shorter.

4 Flex the knees fully (i.e. calves on the thighs) and take the flexed legs in the palms of your hands, with your thumbs over the lower medial sides of the knee joints, and your 3rd and 4th fingers directed down the outsides of the legs towards the greater trochanters.

5 **Without applying any backwards or forwards pressure**, gently abduct both hips simultaneously (Ortolani's manoeuvre).
   - A **normal** hip will abduct fully, the thigh coming to rest on the bed.
   - A **dislocated, reducible** hip will relocate the femoral head into the acetabular fossa during abduction. This action can be felt by the examiner as a clunk, and can often be seen by an observer.
   - A **dislocated, non-reducible** hip will abduct to only about 45°.

6 Now you need to examine for the dislocatable hip (Barlow's manoeuvre).
   - Maintain abduction of each side in turn to stabilise the pelvis while examining the other hip.
   - On the side to be examined, change your grip by moving your thumb higher up the medial thigh.
   - At about 45° abduction, push back with your thumb, attempting to dislocate the femoral head. If the hip is dislocatable, a distinct movement (sometimes called a 'clunk') will be felt as the femoral head rides over the posterior edge of the acetabular fossa.
   - Gently rock the femur between thumb and 3rd and 4th fingers to confirm dislocatability/reducibility.

Hip ultrasound

Some units use hip ultrasound to screen for congenital hip dysplasia. Others may use ultrasound in specific groups of babies (such as those born breech, those with an affected first-degree relative, or with other features of in-utero compression).

Treatment of hip problems

1 **Dislocated, non-reducible** hip — these require orthopaedic consultation. Advise the relevant paediatric/neonatal consultant first.

2 **Dislocated, reducible** and **dislocatable** hips — these may be observed for a few days in hospital. Advise the relevant paediatric consultant, who may wish to feel the hip early. If, by the time of discharge, the hip is still abnormal, it should have firmer splinting in a von Rosen splint, supervised by the orthopaedic department.

3 After discharge, a follow-up appointment should be made for all babies who have had abnormal hips in the neonatal period, **for not more than 3 weeks** following discharge. X-ray at 5–6 months old. Follow up until walking OK.

CHAPTER 26

Maternal infections

Garry Inglis, Mark Davies and David Cartwright

Viral disorders

Hepatitis B

Mothers who are positive for hepatitis B surface antigen (HBsAg) are at risk of passing the virus to their infants (risk 5–20%). The risk is estimated to be between 70% and 90% if they also have the hepatitis B e antigen (HBeAg).

The time of most risk for the infant is the birth process, when the infant comes into contact with maternal blood and secretions. Antenatal transmission is very rare. Infants who acquire hepatitis B have >90% chance of chronic infection.

Prophylaxis

- For babies born to HBsAg-positive mothers, the generally accepted approach is to give the baby hepatitis B immunoglobulin (100 IU, intramuscular, in Australia) as well as the hepatitis B immunisation in the opposite limb. Immunoglobulin should ideally be given before 12 hours of age. This regimen results in >90% protection.
- Before commencing the above schedule, it should be discussed with the parents, or at least the mother, when possible. However, if the mother is unavailable (e.g. after a general anaesthetic), the immunoglobulin should be given anyway. This is just as important as treating pneumonia with antibiotics.
- Serology testing of the infant should not be done before 9 months of age.
- Breastfeeding is not contraindicated.

Immunisation

The most effective way of preventing hepatitis B infection is immunisation prior to exposure to the virus. Routine immunisation in infancy has been introduced in some countries.

- In Australia, this begins at birth and the dose is 5 μg, given by intramuscular injection. Other countries use 10 μg.
- Immunisation should be administered in hospital prior to discharge (when the baby is 'physiologically stable') and preferably in the first 24 hours of life.
  Babies admitted to our intensive care nursery are deemed to be 'physiologically stable' at the time of their discharge/transfer from intensive care. These babies could be going to the postnatal ward, to another hospital, or to the special care nursery. For those admitted to our special care nursery the immunisation will be given when 'physiologically stable' as decided by the medical staff.
- The rate of seroconversion following primary immunisation in children is close to 100%, therefore serology testing is not required.

Note that for babies born in Australia at <32 weeks gestational age (GA), hepatitis B immunisation will not be given until the first general immunisation time at 2 months of age, **except** to those whose mothers are HBsAg-positive for whom hepatitis B vaccination will be given as per the program for term infants.

Some countries adopt a risk-based approach to immunisation, where babies are offered hepatitis B immunisation if they fall into high-risk populations such as certain ethnic groups, or those whose mothers have a history of intravenous drug use.

Hepatitis C virus (HCV)

The risk of vertical transmission from a HCV-infected mother to her baby is approximately 5%. There is inadequate evidence currently available to support the use of prophylactic immunoglobulin for infants born to HCV-infected mothers.

- Breastfeeding is not contraindicated but should be stopped if the mother's nipples are cracked or bleeding.

- There is currently no uniform recommendation for how and when to screen infants born to HCV-positive mothers. Some recommend serology between 6 and 12 months, but specificity is low because passively transferred maternal antibodies can persist until about 18 months. Others delay serology testing until after 18 months. HCV PCR may be available but has been shown to have low sensitivity in the first few months after birth.

Varicella

- Zoster immunoglobulin (ZIG) should be given to any baby whose mother develops varicella up to 7 days before delivery or up to 28 days after delivery.
  - ZIG should be given to the baby as soon after the delivery as possible and must be given within 72 hours.
  - Follow up all babies who are given ZIG. They should be admitted to hospital if any rash develops.
- Intravenous aciclovir should be given:
  - to babies presenting with chickenpox who are unwell (e.g. poor feeding, tachypnoea), whether or not they received ZIG
  - to any high-risk neonate who develops chickenpox and who inadvertently did not receive ZIG prophylaxis or for whom it was delayed beyond 24 hours
  - to immunocompromised neonates who develop chickenpox, including those who are premature or being treated with corticosteroids.
- There is no evidence to support the use of routine aciclovir prophylaxis in conjunction with ZIG and it is not currently recommended in neonates.
- Breastfeeding of infected or exposed babies is encouraged.
- A mother and/or her baby with active vesicles should be isolated from other mothers and babies, but an infected mother does not need to be isolated from her own baby.

[Heuchan A, Isaacs D, on behalf of the Australasian Subgroup in Paediatric Infectious Diseases of the Australasian Society for Infectious Diseases. The management of varicella-zoster virus exposure and infection in pregnancy and the newborn period. Med J Australia 2001;174:288–292.]

Herpes

Neonatal herpes simplex virus (HSV) infection can manifest as mucocutaneous disease, central nervous system (CNS) disease, or disseminated multi-organ disease. The risk of mortality in infected neonates is high and survivors have a high risk of long-term morbidity. Most affected infants will be born to asymptomatic mothers or mothers with no documented history of herpes infection.

- The **risk of transmission** from an infected mother to her vaginally delivered baby is estimated to be <5% for active recurrent genital herpes, and up to 50% for primary infection. For infants delivered by Caesarean section with membranes ruptured for less than 4 hours, the transmission risk is very low.
- All infants born to mothers with **active herpes infection** should be carefully examined and observed for signs of infection.
- Infants born to mothers with **recurrent infection**, and who have **no signs of infection**, are **not** routinely treated with aciclovir.

There are two general approaches to infants born to mothers with primary genital infection.

1. The first approach is to collect swabs within 48 hours of birth from the mouth, conjunctivae, nasopharynx and rectum for HSV PCR (polymerase chain reaction) or culture — if positive then treat with aciclovir.
2. The alternative approach is to treat all babies with aciclovir from birth after collecting swabs as above.

When collecting a swab from a skin lesion, de-roof the lesion and swab from the base.

Any infant who develops clinical evidence of herpes should be treated immediately. If infection is suspected then HSV culture or PCR should be obtained on skin lesion fluid, stool, urine, blood buffy coat and cerebrospinal fluid (CSF).

- Treatment consists of intravenous aciclovir 20 mg/kg/dose every 8 hours for 14 days (mucocutaneous disease only) or 21 days (disseminated or CNS disease).

Human immunodeficiency virus (HIV)

HIV screening in pregnancy is routine in some places. Pregnant women known to be HIV-positive should be treated during pregnancy and labour. Caesarean delivery before membrane rupture has been shown to reduce the risk of transmission.

- Babies born to HIV-positive mothers should be treated with zidovudine (2 mg/kg every 6 hours orally) for the first 6 weeks of life. This has been shown to reduce the risk of transmission by about two-thirds.
- HIV screening of the infant by DNA PCR (polymease chain reaction) should be done in the first few days of life and repeated at 1–2 and 4 months.
- In developed countries breastfeeding should be discouraged because of the risk of transmission.

Syphilis

- Infants born to mothers with a history of adequately treated syphilis (who have not been reinfected) usually require no specific treatment but must be evaluated for evidence of infection: examine the infant carefully and check antibody titre (RPR, rapid plasma reagin test).
    - If the titre is 4 times higher than the mother's then treat.
- All babies born to mothers with a history of syphilis should be followed up to document a negative RPR.

Infants should definitely be treated if their mothers were:

- not treated or inadequately treated
- treated with a non-penicillin drug
- treated less than 4 weeks prior to delivery.

In practice the adequacy of a mother's prior treatment can be difficult to establish, and you can rarely be confident the mother has not been reinfected since the last course of treatment. Therefore, under these circumstances it is safer to treat all babies.

Treatment is intravenous benzylpenicillin 50 mg/kg/dose twice a day for 10 days, or intramuscular procaine penicillin 50 mg/kg daily for 10 days.

CHAPTER 27

Audiology

Garry Inglis

Routine audiology screening for all babies, ideally just prior to discharge from hospital, was introduced in Queensland in 2004. Prior to the introduction of screening, the average age at detection of permanent hearing impairment was 30 months. It is hoped that screening will allow earlier detection and therefore improved speech and language development in those affected. Keep in mind that screening will not usually detect mild hearing impairment.

- Babies become eligible for screening at 34 weeks gestational age.
- Screening is done using automated auditory brainstem response (AABR).
- Babies who have risk factors for progressive or delayed-onset hearing loss are referred for diagnostic audiology in the first year (see list below).

Other health authorities may use targeted surveillance, in which infants with certain risk factors are referred for audiology.

Risk factors include:

1 A family history of permanent hearing loss in childhood in first-degree relatives (this does not include acquired conditions such as recurrent ear infections or trauma).
2 Syndromes associated with hearing loss (e.g. Down syndrome, CHARGE).
3 Birth weight (e.g. in Queensland, ≤1500 g).
4 Bacterial meningitis.
5 Severe perinatal asphyxia.
6 Craniofacial anomalies (excluding simple pre-auricular tags and cleft lip).

7. Significant hyperbilirubinaemia (e.g. in Queensland, ≥450 μmol/L at ≥37 weeks; ≥340 μmol/L <37 weeks).
8. Congenital infection (cytomegalovirus, herpes, rubella, toxoplasmosis, syphilis).
9. Professional concern about hearing.
10. Prolonged respiratory support (e.g. in Queensland, ≥5 days).
11. Other reason for prolonged admission to a neonatal intensive care unit.
12. Parental or caregiver concern about hearing or delayed development.

Risk factors 1–10 are those used for diagnostic audiology referral in Queensland. Note that the use of aminoglycoside antibiotics is generally not considered a criterion for referral in the absence of other risk factors.

CHAPTER 28

Immunisation

David Cartwright

> **!** It is important to refer to your local immunisation schedule.

- Preterm babies should be immunised according to their chronological age, 'provided that they are well and that there are no contraindications to vaccination', with the exception that the option is given in the *Australian Immunisation Handbook* for babies born at less than 32 weeks of gestation to receive their first hepatitis B immunisation with the normal first general immunisation at 2 months of age.

  All babies with this degree of immaturity should receive a 'booster' hepatitis B immunisation at 12 months of age, whether or not they received one at birth.
- The other standard immunisations at 2 months (in Australia) are for diphtheria, whooping cough and tetanus (DTPa), pneumococcus (7-valent), polio (intramuscular) and *Haemophilus influenzae* type B (Hib).

  These are presented in various combinations in different states (Queensland has 3 injections: Hib–HepB, DTPa–IPOL and Prevenar). [IPOL — polio; Prevenar — pneumococcus.]
- The *Australian Immunisation Handbook* states:
  — 'When PedvaxHIB is used in an extremely preterm baby (<28 weeks gestation or <1500 g birth weight), an additional dose of vaccine should be given at

6 months of age (i.e. doses should be given at 2, 4, 6 and 12 months of age)'

and additionally

— 'All preterm babies born at less than 28 weeks' gestation or with chronic lung disease should be offered the 7-valent pneumococcal conjugate vaccine at 2, 4 and 6 months of age with a fourth dose at 12 months of age, and a 23-valent pneumococcal polysaccharide vaccine booster at 4 to 5 years of age'.

- Your local authority will have a list of ethnic groups who are at higher risk of tuberculosis because of local family associations or movement between home and their country of origin. Babies born into these families should receive BCG vaccination.

CHAPTER 29

Vitamin K

David Cartwright

Vitamin K is given to newborn infants to prevent haemorrhagic disease of the newborn (HDN), which occurs in about 1 in 10,000 births. Bleeding can occur in the first week of life or up to a month or two of age; devastating intracranial bleeding is common with late-onset HDN. Babies who are breastfed are at highest risk. Almost all cases can be prevented by a single intramuscular injection (IM) dose of vitamin K.

- The National Health and Medical Research Council (NHMRC) of Australia recommends that all babies get an IM dose of 1 mg (0.1 mL) of Konakion MM at birth.
- The IM dose is stressed as the preferred option for reliability and compliance. However, parents can elect to have the vitamin K treatment administered orally as three 2 mg (0.2 mL) doses of Konakion MM. These doses are given at birth, at the time of newborn screening (3 to 5 days), and at 4 weeks.
- The NHMRC recommendations stress that 'the advantage of the intramuscular injection is it requires no subsequent dosage to be administered. The advantage of the oral administration in three doses is that it is non-invasive and that, if 100% compliance is achieved, it may be almost as effective as intramuscular administration'.
- The guidelines also stress the need for parents to receive written information during the antenatal period about the importance of vitamin K and the options of intramuscular or oral treatments.

- The guidelines also stress that child-health workers and parents should be aware that unexplained bleeding or bruising in infants is uncommon and should be promptly investigated and treated. Information on unexplained bleeding is recommended for inclusion in the general information provided to parents during the antenatal period.
- Whilst a single, flawed, study showed an association between IM vitamin K (in a preparation that is no longer used) and childhood cancer, it has now been shown in multiple subsequent studies that this association **does not exist**.

CHAPTER 30

Withdrawal of treatment

Mark Davies and David Cartwright

General principles

In certain circumstances it is considered appropriate to withdraw life support from an infant, or to not initiate life support. This will always be done with close collaboration between the consultant responsible for that baby's care, the nursing and social work staff, and the baby's parents; embracing the principles established at consensus conferences in New South Wales in 1986, 1989 and 1998, and the findings of the latest consensus conference held in Australia (published in 2006). [Lui K et al. Perinatal care at the borderlines of viability: a consensus statement based on a NSW and ACT consensus workshop. Med J Australia 2006;185(9):495–500.]

- Consideration must be given to the interests and wellbeing of the infant.
- The initiation or the prolongation of treatment is not necessarily in the best interests of the infant.
- The opinion of parents as to the best interests of the infant must be respected and accounted for.
- Society has the right to intervene when parents' decisions are not clearly in the best interests of the infant.
- Resources are finite. There may be competing financial claims which are as vital to human life as is neonatal intensive care.
- Parents must be informed and consulted about all medical treatment or non-treatment regarding their newborn child.

- Appropriate follow-up is essential, including support for parents of disabled survivors and community services for such infants.

Non-initiation of life support

- Initiation of life support is inappropriate in infants born with lethal non-correctable malformations (such as anencephaly and confirmed trisomy 13 or 18).
  If possible, this eventuality should be discussed with the parents before birth.
- There exists a discretionary zone ('grey zone') in neonatal practice. Within this zone, after considered discussion between parent and specialist caregivers, it would be acceptable and reasonable medical practice to not initiate life support for a newborn.
  Informed discussion should commence before the birth.
- The location of the 'grey zone' boundaries are at 25^{+6} and 23^{+0} weeks.
  - At 26^{+0} weeks and above, there is indication to treat unless there are exceptional circumstances.
  - Below 23^{+0} weeks, resuscitation and active treatment are not appropriate.
- The decision whether to initiate treatment or not within the 'grey zone' will depend on the wishes of the parents and other factors such as the condition of the baby at birth and past obstetric history. Under these circumstances counselling should always include the option of not starting resuscitation and active treatment, and the potential consequences of active intervention.
- These 'grey zone' boundaries, it is appreciated, may be inappropriate in areas with no neonatal intensive care facilities and where transport may be impractical.

Withdrawal of treatment

It is reasonable and acceptable practice to withdraw treatment under certain circumstances. Where an infant is dependent on medical treatment for survival, it is reasonable and accepted practice to withdraw such treatment, after considered discussion between parent and specialist caregiver, in any one of the following situations:

1. There is a substantial probability of major disability if that treatment were to continue (very little chance of normal outcome).
2. Death is inevitable and imminent regardless of that treatment (i.e. treatment is futile).
3. Continued treatment cannot relieve pain and suffering believed to be intolerable.

CHAPTER 31

Death

Mark Davies and David Cartwright

Actions at death of a baby

When a baby dies:

- Ensure that a formal note is inserted in the chart indicating death and the assessment made to ascertain this.
- Collect blood on a neonatal screening card (if baby has not had one collected already); label as post-mortem.
- Ensure that the events leading up to the death are adequately and clearly described in the chart notes.
- Discuss post-mortem examination (PM) with the parents before they leave the hospital — make a note in the chart as to whether the parents agree to a PM or do not want a PM.
- Written consent from a parent is now standard procedure (and a legal requirement in many places, e.g. Queensland) before proceeding with any PM.
- The death certificate should be completed by, at the latest, the next working day.
- Nursing staff should make arrangements for appropriate material to be given to the parents, and for social work follow-up. The parents should be offered an appointment with the consultant neonatologist who cared for the baby.

Unexplained neonatal death

In the event of an unexplained neonatal death, the results of investigations done on the following specimens may help with determining a possible cause of death and aid in counselling parents about future pregnancies.

Take the specimens as soon after death as possible (with parental consent) and discuss with pathology/metabolic medicine and genetics later.

Specimens to collect

1. Blood on a neonatal screening card (label card as post-mortem specimen).
2. Urine (freeze).
3. Chromosomes, DNA (2 mL of blood in an EDTA tube).
4. A whole baby X-ray (babygram).

All of these are achievable without the need for autopsy — and the first three are not likely to be successfully collected if the baby goes to autopsy.

The coroner

Whilst the provisions of Coroners' Acts will vary from state to state and across countries, the following circumstances will usually require a death to be reported to the coroner:

- the identity of the baby is unknown
- the baby is in care
- the death was violent, unnatural or occurred under suspicious circumstances
- a death certificate cannot be written
- the death was not reasonably expected to be the outcome of a health-related procedure.

If in doubt, talk to the coroner.

CHAPTER 32

Outcome statistics

Mark Davies

The following statistics for survival and morbidity relate to outcomes of interest at the time of hospital discharge.

The outcomes shown are for babies born at the Royal Brisbane and Women's Hospital (RBWH), from 2000 to 2005 inclusive. These data, while specific for the RBWH, will give ball park numbers that will be of some use when counselling parents.

Survival

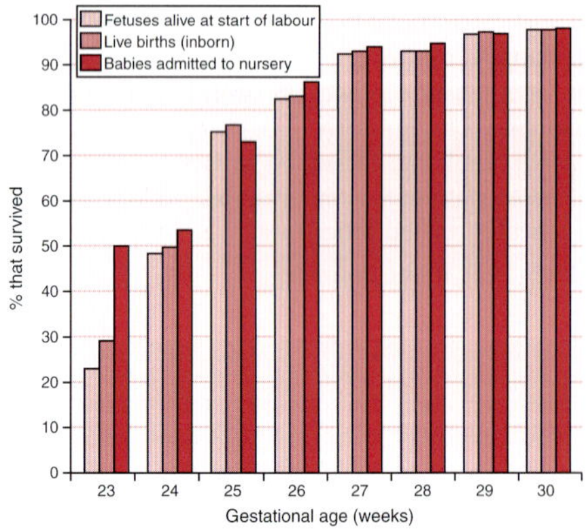

Figure 32.1 Survival statistics

Morbidity

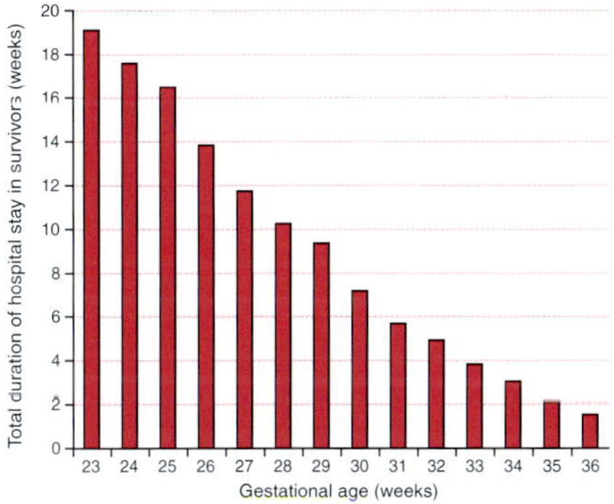

Figure 32.2 Duration of total hospital stay in babies surviving to discharge

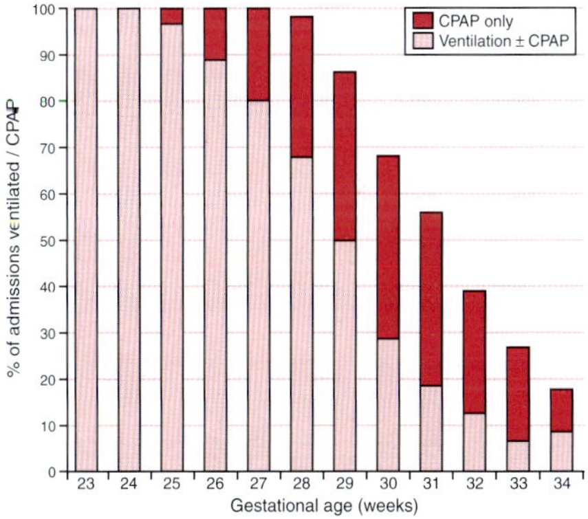

Figure 32.3 Proportion of babies admitted who had respiratory support

CPAP = continuous positive airway pressure

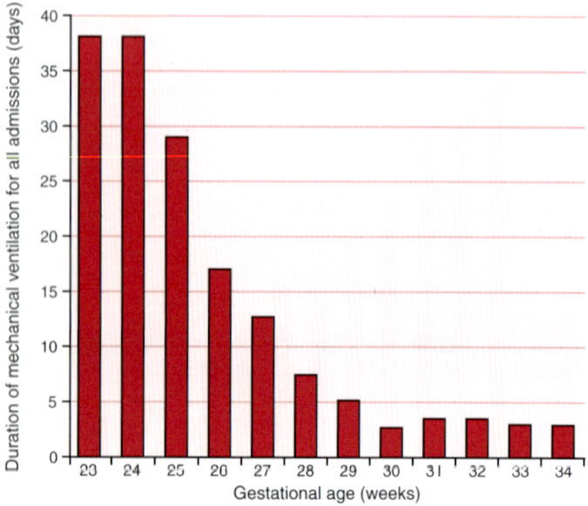

Figure 32.4 Duration of mechanical ventilation for all admissions

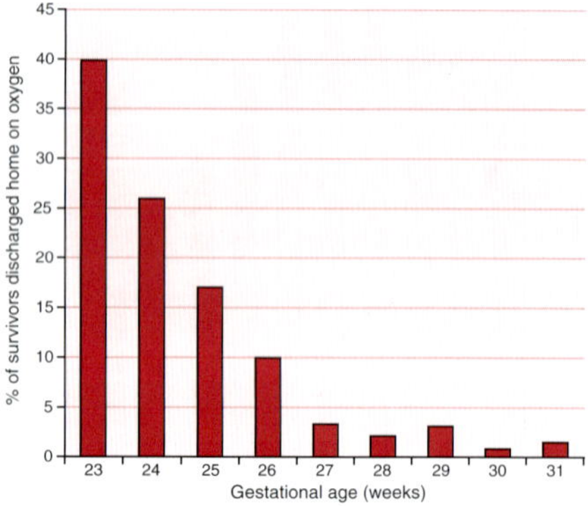

Figure 32.5 Proportion of survivors who went home on oxygen therapy

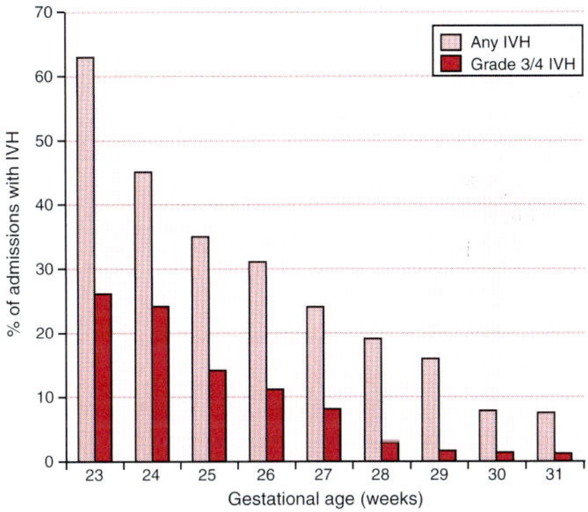

Figure 32.6 Proportion of all admissions who had intraventricular haemorrhage (IVH)

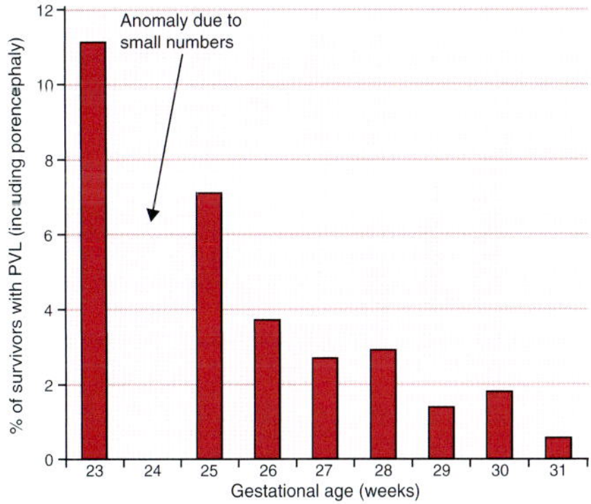

Figure 32.7 Proportion of all survivors who had periventricular leucomalacia (PVL)

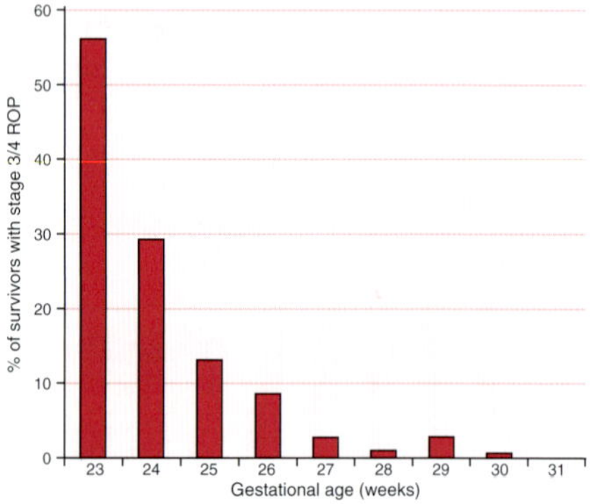

Figure 32.8 Proportion of all survivors who had severe retinopathy of prematurity (ROP)

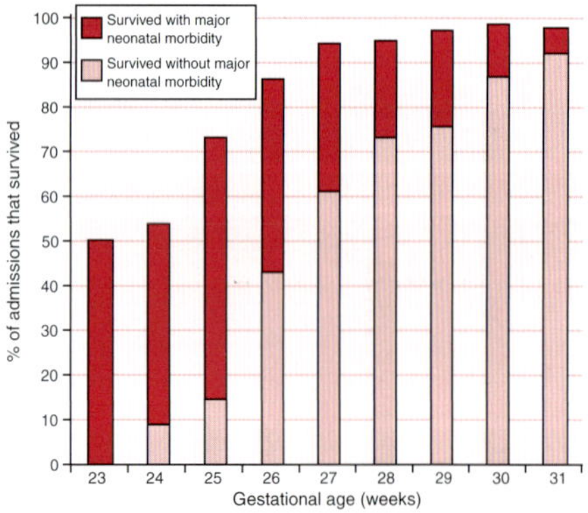

Figure 32.9 Proportion of all survivors with major neonatal morbidity
Major neonatal morbidity = oxygen at 36 weeks, or definite necrotising enterocolitis (NEC), or retinopathy of prematurity (ROP) stage 3 or 4, or intraventricular haemorrhage (IVH) grade 3 or 4, or periventricular leukomalacia (PVL), or porencephalic cyst, or hydrocephalus

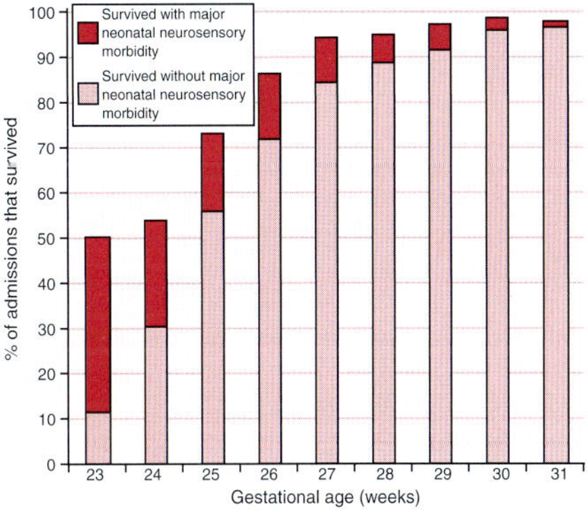

Figure 32.10 Proportion of all survivors with major neonatal neurosensory morbidity

Major neonatal neurosensory morbidity = retinopathy of prematurity (ROP) stage ≥3, or intraventricular haemorrhage (IVH) grade 3 or 4, or periventricular leukomalacia (PVL), or porencephalic cyst, or hydrocephalus

Long-term outcome

Preterm infants are at risk for adverse neurodevelopmental outcome. This may include non-specific developmental delay, cerebral palsy (CP), intellectual deficit, deafness and blindness.

The following data are derived from combining the data from a few recent studies and follow-up data from the RBWH. They are a rough guide only: the confidence intervals around them are wide. The following definitions for the levels of disability are an example of those used:

- moderate disability — Developmental Quotient between 2 and 3 standard deviations below the mean; deaf; moderate CP (walks with aids)
- severe disability — Developmental Quotient more than 3 standard deviations below the mean; blind; severe CP (unable to walk).

Gestational age (weeks)	% moderate/severe disability
23	~55
24	~35
25	~30
26	~25
27	~20
28	~15
29	<10
30	<10
31	<5
32	<5
33	<5

CHAPTER 33

The ready reckoner

Mark Davies

The following pages contain information useful when admitting a sick infant to intensive care.

The tables contain information (by infant weight) on the size of endotracheal tubes (ETTs) and umbilical lines to use; how far to insert them; and common drug and infusion doses.

Note that the insertion lengths of umbilical catheters are given in cm from the plane of the abdominal wall.

> **!** The information is a guide only. All tubes and lines must be checked radiologically for correct placement, and drug doses and infusions checked and titrated to the needs of individual infants.

Table 33.1 Approximate 50th centile birth weights at various gestational ages (combined male and female)

Gestational age (weeks)	Weight (g)	Gestational age (weeks)	Weight (g)
22	487	29	1285
23	585	30	1450
24	684	32	1832
25	786	34	2276
26	893	36	2756
27	1009	38	3198
28	1138	40	3506

Baby's weight (g)	ETT size	Tape oral ETT at lip (cm)	Dose of Survanta 4 mL/kg	UAC & UVC size (FG)	UAC insertion length (cm)	UVC insertion length (cm)	mL/hr total fluids if total daily fluids = 60 mL/kg/day	Dose of penicillin 60 mg/kg	Dose of gentamicin 2.5 mg/kg	10 mL/kg = (mL)	Bolus dose of either morphine or midazolam (mg)	Dose (in mg) of morphine or midazolam in 50 mL syringe for infusion 0.5 mL/hr = 10 μg/kg/hr	Dose (in mg) of dopamine or dobutamine in 50 mL syringe for infusion 1 mL/hr = 10 μg/kg/min
500	2.5	6.0	2	3.5	10.5	6.4	1.3	30	1.3	5	0.05	0.5	15
550	2.5	6.0	2.2	3.5	10.7	6.4	1.4	33	1.4	6	0.06	0.55	17
600	2.5	6.0	2.4	3.5	10.8	6.5	1.5	36	1.5	6	0.06	0.6	18
650	2.5	6.5	2.6	3.5	11.0	6.6	1.6	39	1.6	7	0.07	0.65	20
700	2.5	6.5	2.8	3.5	11.1	6.7	1.8	42	1.8	7	0.07	0.7	21
750	2.5	6.5	3	3.5	11.3	6.7	1.9	45	1.9	8	0.08	0.75	23
800	2.5	6.5	3.2	3.5	11.4	6.8	2.0	48	2.0	8	0.08	0.8	24
850	2.5	6.5	3.4	3.5	11.6	6.9	2.1	51	2.1	9	0.09	0.85	26
900	2.5	7.0	3.6	3.5	11.7	7.0	2.3	54	2.3	9	0.09	0.9	27
950	2.5	7.0	3.8	3.5	11.9	7.0	2.4	57	2.4	10	0.10	0.95	29

Table 33.2a Ready reckoner for infant weights of 500–950 g

ETT = endotracheal tube; UAC = umbilical arterial catheter; UVC = umbilical venous catheter

Baby's weight (g)	ETT size	Tape oral ETT at lip (cm)	Dose of Survanta 4 mL/kg	UAC & UVC size (FG)	UAC insertion length (cm)	UVC insertion length (cm)	mL/hr total fluids if total daily fluids = 60 mL/kg/day	Dose of penicillin 60 mg/kg	Dose of gentamicin 2.5 mg/kg	10 mL/kg = (mL)	Bolus dose of either morphine or midazolam (mg)	Dose (in mg) of morphine or midazolam in 50 mL syringe for infusion 0.5 mL/hr = 10 μg/kg/hr	Dose (in mg) of dopamine or dobutmine in 50 mL syringe for infusion 1 mL/hr = 10 μg/kg/min
1000	2.5/3.0	7.0	4	3.5	12.2	7.1	2.5	60	2.5	0	0.10	1.0	30
1100	2.5/3.0	7.0	4.4	3.5	12.5	7.3	2.8	66	2.8	1	0.11	1.1	33
1200	2.5/3.0	7.0	4.8	3.5	12.7	7.4	3.0	72	3.0	2	0.12	1.2	36
1300	3.0	7.5	5.2	3.5	13.0	7.6	3.3	78	3.3	3	0.13	1.3	39
1400	3.0	7.5	5.6	3.5/5	13.2	7.7	3.5	84	3.5	4	0.14	1.4	42
1500	3.0	7.5	6	5	13.5	7.9	3.8	90	3.8	5	0.15	1.5	45
1600	3.0	7.5	6.4	5	13.7	8.0	4.0	96	4.0	6	0.16	1.6	48
1700	3.0	7.5	6.8	5	14.0	8.2	4.3	102	4.3	7	0.17	1.7	51
1800	3.0	8.0	7.2	5	14.2	8.3	4.5	108	4.5	8	0.18	1.8	54
1900	3.0	8.0	7.6	5	14.5	8.5	4.8	114	4.8	9	0.19	1.9	57

Table 33.2b Ready reckoner for infant weights of 1000–1900 g

ETT = endotracheal tube; UAC = umbilical arterial catheter; UVC = umbilical venous catheter

Baby's weight (g)	ETT size	Tape oral ETT at lip (cm)	Dose of Survanta 4 mL/kg	UAC & UVC size (FG)	UAC insertion length (cm)	UVC insertion length (cm)	mL/hr total fluids if total daily fluids = 60 mL/kg/day	Dose of penicillin 60 mg/kg	Dose of gentamicin 2.5 mg/kg	10 mL/kg = (mL)	Bolus dose of either morphine or midazolam (mg)	Dose (in mg) of morphine or midazolam in 50 mL syringe for infusion 0.5 mL/hr = 10 µg/kg/hr	Dose (in mg) of dopamine or dobutmine in 50 mL syringe for infusion 1 mL/hr = 10 µg/kg/min
2000	3.0	8.0	8	5	14.7	8.6	5.0	120	5.0	20	0.20	2.0	60
2200	3.0/3.5	8.0	8.8	5	15.2	8.9	5.5	132	5.5	22	0.22	2.2	66
2400	3.0/3.5	8.5	9.6	5	15.7	9.2	6.0	144	6.0	24	0.24	2.4	72
2600	3.0/3.5	8.5	10.4	5	16.2	9.5	6.5	156	6.5	26	0.26	2.6	78
2800	3.5	9.0	11.2	5	16.7	9.8	7.0	168	7.0	28	0.28	2.8	84
3000	3.5	9.0	12	5	17.2	10.1	7.5	180	7.5	30	0.30	3.0	90
3200	3.5	9.0	12.8	5	17.7	10.4	8.0	192	8.0	32	0.32	3.2	96
3400	3.5	9.5	13.6	5	18.2	10.7	8.5	204	8.5	34	0.34	3.4	102
3600	3.5	9.5	14.4	5	18.7	11.0	9.0	216	9.0	36	0.36	3.6	108
3800	3.5	10.0	15.2	5	19.2	11.3	9.5	228	9.5	38	0.38	3.8	114
4000	3.5/4.0	10.0	16	5	19.7	11.6	10.0	240	10.0	40	0.40	4.0	120

Table 33.2c Ready reckoner for infant weights of 2000–4000 g

ETT = endotracheal tube; UAC = umbilical arterial catheter; UVC = umbilical venous catheter

Index

E

I

N

O

R

T

U

V